Disclaimer

The material in this book is presented for informational purposes only and not intended for treatment or diagnosis of any disease. Please consult with a qualified health professional for any ailment discussed or mentioned herein. The author and publisher take no responsibility for the use or misuse of any information presented in this work.

THE BEST NATURAL SPORTS MEDICINE BOOK EVER

ISBN 1-892264-07-2

TIMELESS VOYAGER PRESS
PO Box 6678
Santa Barbara, CA 93160
1-800-576-8463

Covers and book development by Bruce Stephen Holms

Timeless Voyager Press

THE BEST NATURAL SPORTS MEDICINE BOOK EVER

Natural Supplements and Exercise
for Healing Sports Related Injuries

William Wong, N.D., Ph.D.

Formatted and Edited by
Bruce Stephen Holms

TABLE OF CONTENTS

Acknowledgments
• • • • • •

To Professor Dr. Enrico A. Moore Ph.D., Sc.D., and Martial Arts Grandmaster (Soke) for your dedication to and advancement of Sports Medicine and the Martial Arts. Your strength and conviction in the face of adversity will light the way for many.

Publisher Acknowledgments

•• •• ••

The publisher wishes to thank Adam Holms for posing in the many exercise photographs. Thanks also to the Cathedral Oaks Athletic Club in Santa Barbara, CA for allowing Adam to use their facilities and incredible exercise equipment.

Special thanks to Ann Holms for her formatting and editing skills, and Linda White for her thorough first draft editing.

Chapter 1
Why Natural Sports Medicine?
● ● ● ● ● ●

Why a book on the natural treatment of sports injuries? Well, there are an estimated one and a half million sports injuries a year in the US alone. It's not just school athletes that account for the many injuries. Kids playing little league, soccer, gymnastics, or peewee football are suffering the same injuries as the grown-ups. Teens and twenty-somethings expressing the speed and vibrancy of their youth in sport, dance and exercise are going overboard with the "extremeness" of their activity. Thirty and forty something's are trying to keep up with the younger folks to prove they still can, and suffering the consequences. Fifty and sixty-year-olds, noting the loss of strength and ability, are getting hurt attempting TV exercise programs or getting back to their old sports. Our bodies crave movement! Our ambitions for that movement though oftentimes need a little tempering or a large dose of a reality check.

The long and the short of it is that generations are moving, playing, and doing as has never been seen before! Two facts need to be known here.

1 Most sports injuries are mild to moderate. This means that the boo boo is not bad enough to need surgery, casts, or extensive rehab.

2 Most sports injuries are over treated or under treated. MDs frequently use cortisone to treat minor injuries, which can cause everything from tissue death to osteoporosis. Surgery is often advised for minor tears of muscles or ligaments. Why? Well, orthopedists are surgeons first and foremost and, well, they have bills to pay too. (Besides, what do you care – you've got good insurance!) It's either too much treatment or "walk it off and be a man!" type of cave man football coach advice.

Americans need to know that the innocent painkillers we take for granted are real killers. According to the *Wall Street Journal,* twenty thousand people die in the US each year from aspirin, ibuprofen, and acetaminophen. In the UK, Tylenol is sold only by the dose because so many have died unintentionally from kidney failure.

To those used to Allopathic (conventional medicine) treatment of sports injuries, natural medicine's care of those injuries sounds odd ball or out of place. Natural treatments have been used in sports medicine since the days of the first Olympics of Greece 3000 years ago! Natural medicine has been employed to reduce and rehabilitate sports and martial arts injuries in the orient for 5000 years that we know of! Natural medicine makes constant strides, employing the newest electronic technology and knowledge on performance nutrition adding it to the ancient armamentum it contains. Historically speaking, the oddball thing is the trend over the last 175 years to treat sports injuries exclusively with drugs, surgery and physical therapy. (Allopathic medicine is only that many years old).

For those athletes wishing to avoid the surgeons' knife, this book is for you. For parents wanting non-toxic care for the strains and sprains of young players, this book is for you. For thirty something's and forty something's plus, getting beaten up trying to keep up with the young studs, this book is for you. For seniors who are at a loss as to what to do for exercise and activity or are suffering the aches and injuries of over sold exercise programs not even fit for the young, this book is for you. We will cover the most common injuries had in sports, dance and exercise; their evaluation, reduction and rehabilitation. We will learn when the knife and drugs are indicated and we will learn of the options to surgery and drugs. Throughout, our goal will be what Professor William Chisolm so aptly taught us in basic sports medicine at Brooklyn College: The restoration of Full Function, Full Strength, and Pain Free Full Range of Motion.

NOTES

NOTES

Chapter 2
Injury Recovery: Its Nutritional Demands
● ● ● ● ● ●

First and foremost in healing, we need to speed the process by feeding the body the building blocks it needs to reconstruct the damaged tissue. Sports medicine and athletic training have for years ignored the nutritional aspects of rehabilitation. It's not our fault really; sports medicine follows where physical medicine leads. In this country, orthopedists and physiatrists have no good literature available on the feeding of rebuilding tissues. Since nutrition is not a subject taught in medical school, most in rehabilitation have tended to ignore it as unnecessary. Fortunately, medicine elsewhere has not.

Look to see what veterinary medicine is doing with nutrition and you'll see where human nutrition will be in 30 years. Everything from Vitamin C to Glucosamine to MSM first came out of veterinary medicine. It's sad really. Dr. Kassimire Funk may have first discovered vitamins in 1913, but the application of that knowledge to the human end of the mammalian species has taken most of the last century to be realized. Vets know an astounding amount about information on the nutritional needs of their patients. Yet, that information has taken years to filter down to human medicine.

In Europe, especially central and eastern Europe where nutritional science is a more integral part of healing, there is a different outlook on illness and injury. In our country, the medical system does not make money unless a patient gets sick and stays sick. In most of the rest of the world, society loses money if a person gets sick and stays sick. The emphasis, therefore, has been on getting the patient up, back on his/her feet, and functioning as well as possible in as short a time as possible, keeping costs to a minimum. This is especially true in professional sports medicine.

At the fall of the Iron Curtain, Eastern Europe was 20 to 30 years ahead of the Western curve in sports medicine and physical education. With the flow of their physicians, trainers, and coaches to the West, we are now learning that their techniques of conditioning, training, and rehabilitation were superior to ours in terms of producing spectacular results in a short time. Token evidence of their superiority is seen by the fact that the US Olympic Weight lifting Coach was Rumania's National coach, and the Exercise Physiologist in charge of conditioning for the US Marshals Service was a trainer for the elite Soviet Special Forces.

If we combine the knowledge held in veterinary medicine with the techniques and methods of the old eastern block, we will come up with a superior method of getting our athletes back on line in record time with a more fully rounded and complete development. Let's get to the basics, and, to do that, we need a brief review of Histology - the science of living tissue.

There are three types of tissue:

1 **Epithelial Tissue**. This consists of skin, eyes, internal organs (especially the reproductive organs and glands), and muscle. In some classification systems, muscle is its own tissue, but because muscle and epithelial tissue arise from the same embryonic tissue – the mesenchyme – and because it contains the same mineral building block, I include it as epithelial tissue.

2 **Connective Tissue**. This is made up of fascia, ligaments, bones, cartilage, and blood vessels. We will divide connective tissue into soft and hard as each needs different nutrients to form its matrix.

3 **Nervous Tissue**. This consists of the brain and nerves.[1]

Each type of tissue depends on different nutrients to form its matrix. Everyone should know that bone is made up of calcium, magnesium, and phosphorus. Soft connective tissue (i.e., fascia, cartilage, and blood vessels) is made from "sulfated mucopolyaccharide", so its primary mineral component is sulfur.[2]

Epithelial tissue is based on zinc while nervous tissue is not primarily mineral-based but is 60% to 70% cholesterol in the form of lipo/proteins. The next time someone calls you a fathead thank them; they've just paid your brain a compliment.

For decades in the west, it was assumed that our diet was complete enough to provide all of the nutrients necessary to maintain and rebuild tissue. Soil depletion and Agra business growing techniques have resulted in today's food being mostly devoid of mineral nutrition.[3] This lack means we must provide a constant supply of the building blocks needed to maintain tissue. Moreover, during times of recovery from heavy training or injury, we need to provide an abundant supply of tissue nutrients to keep micro trauma from developing into macro trauma and to speed the healing of tissue.

All right, let's get to brass tacks; what specifically do I recommend feeding an athlete recovering from injury? Let's take it tissue by tissue.

Epithelial Tissue. The mineral basis here is zinc, and the need is for 50mg most training days. During injury, especially extensive injury to soft tissue, up the dose to 100mg for the duration of rehab. Zinc is only toxic in doses above 300mg a day and only if taken for extended periods. There is much ado today about having to balance zinc with copper. Yes, for every 100mg of zinc we need 3mg of copper, but we in the States are far from being copper deficient. Most of us have copper pipes in our homes, and this fact alone provides us with the 3mg we need. If there is an imbalance, the excess does not rest on the zinc side; we hardly have any true dietary sources of zinc. To get our needed dose of zinc, we would have to eat a bushel of whole wheat, a side of beef, or a basket full of oysters. The old wives' tale about oysters being aphrodisiac arises from the experience of zinc-deficient men eating oysters and suddenly having their prostates work again, churning out semen. Zinc is the reason why semen is white and is essential for the production of testosterone and the production of sperm.

You will also notice that in terms of dose I said "needed" instead of required (referring to the RDA guidelines of the FDA). The National Academy of Science has been trying for years to have the government change the way they determine the RDA. Here's how the FDA figures out how much of what nutrients you need: A lab mouse of some 1 or 2 ounces is taken and starved of a particular nutrient until it develops a macro-deficiency disease. In other words, if they are looking at Vitamin C, the scientists will ignore the bleeding gums, the hair falling out, the connective tissue degeneration. It's not until the little mouse gets full-blown scurvy that they take notice. The eggheads in the lab then go back to the dose they were administering before it got full blown sick and they add five units of measure to that figure and presto – you have the RDA! I put it to you that the physiological processes of a growing or full grown human are greater than those of a 2-ounce lab mouse! But back to facts and figures.

For the muscular portion of epithelial tissue, we must also include 1 gram of protein per kilo of bodyweight. Some athletes depending on their build, their training, or the demands of their sport may need less; archers vs. football linemen for example. Many trainers out there who are working with bodybuilding protocols instead of true strength training protocols are stuck in a "we need a gram of protein or more per pound of bodyweight" rut. This formula has never been true. It was invented to sell bodybuilding supplements! That much protein creates a huge ammonia load on the kidneys, leading to a condition known as glomerulosclerosis (fibrosis of the kidney). Kidney troubles are one of the leading killers of athletes and body builders – why create one of the conditions for kidney damage?

Connective Tissue. For soft connective tissue the answer is simple: organic sulfur in the form of MSM is needed to the tune of from 500 to 1500mg daily depending on the location and extent of the injury. For example: lumbo dorsal fascia tear - 500 to 1000mg a day vs. cartilage tear, herniation, or fracture - 1500mg. This substance is the brick that forms connective tissue; now for the cement - Vitamin C. Two capsules twice a day.

That will provide the sulfur; now for the mucopolysaccharide. Use glucosamine HCl (the HCl is absorbed better and works faster than the glucosamine sulfate), and chondroitin sulfate to the tune of 750 to 1600mg daily, again depending on the extent and location of the injury. These provide the joints with the wherewithal to recoat worn smooth cartilage.

In cases of hard connective tissue injury the body needs: 1000mg of calcium, 600mg of magnesium, phosphorus, and the bone builders vitamins D and K. We need not provide the phosphorus as most athletes drink cola and sodas where phosphorus is found in abundance.

Magnesium all by itself is needed for the function of 2600 of the body's more than 3000 enzymes, many of which are involved in healing. Magnesium is responsible for muscular relaxation. Spasm cannot occur if tissue magnesium concentrations are high enough (i.e., around 2000mg a day). Magnesium is safe. Allopathic (conventional) physicians order doses of 446,729 mg (or 1 gallon) of magnesium citrate, (the most absorbable form of magnesium), before colonoscopy without any more ill effects than the runs.

Enzymes

Now we come to the most important part of nutritional healing, enzymes. Again in the States the medical education concerning enzymes is non-existent; so, medical science here doesn't know what medical science elsewhere has been doing with enzymes for 40+ years. Let's first give you some history.

The year was 1912: Scottish physician, Dr. John Beard noticed that pancreatic cancer patients produced little or no pancreatic enzymes. He began feeding these patients extracts of fresh pancreas and in many of his patients the death sentence of pancreatic cancer was lifted. However, not knowing how to stabilize his extract, the results of others with enzymes proved erratic.

In the 1920's –1970's, Dr. Max Wolf was the world's foremost researcher in enzymology. Dr. Wolf was an MD who also held seven PhDs. He taught medical school at Fordham and did research with Dr. Helen Benetiz at Columbia University. Dr. Wolf practiced medicine as an OBGYN and wrote the first medical textbook on endocrinology in the 1920s. While studying hormones, he became fascinated with the other regulatory mechanism of the body – enzymes. We tend to think of these critters solely as agents of digestion, but that is only one of thousands and thousands of actions that enzymes perform in the body. Of all the enzymes, the protein cleaving enzymes are the most important to the regulation of physiology.

Four Functions: In brief, the four most important functions of the protein-eating enzymes are these:

One. The anti-inflammatory function enzymes are the first line of defense against inflammation. The body's cortico steroids are the second. All inflammation is caused by Circulating Immune Complexes (CIC) created by the immune system. For example, if an athlete has hurt his knee, the immune system creates this CIC protein and tags it to go to the effected knee. (The Nobel Prize in biology for '99 was won by the fellow who figured out how these proteins get tagged.) There the CIC creates inflammation - redness, swelling, and pain - as a protective splinting mechanism. Aspirin, ibuprofen, and the other NSAID drugs, both COX I and COX II, work by keeping the body from making CICs. At first glance this action may sound just fine – until you remember that the kidneys are run by CICs and that the intestinal lining is maintained by CICs. Not all CICs are bad but these medications can't tell the difference. So they stop all Circulating Immune Complexes. Twenty thousand Americans die each year because these drugs can't tell the difference. Another 100,000 wind up hospitalized because of these side effects or with the liver toxicity they create.[4]

Proteolytic enzymes, on the other hand, are specific lock and key mechanisms. They look for exogenous proteins, proteins that are not what they consider to be part of the body's TRUE structure, and eat them! Just like Pacman eating the little dots. The CICs that create inflammation are differentiated from the ones that maintain visceral function; enzymes leave those alone while chomping down on the bad CICs. Dr. Wolf discovered this in the 1930s![5]

Two. The second function of protein eating enzymes is to act as an Anti-Fibrotic. Enzymes are what the body uses to control the part of its healing mechanism that deals with fibrin. Fibrin is connective tissue that the body deposits into a wound or injury to act as a matrix through which the healing takes place. Let's use this simple example. When you are young and cut your finger, the wound heals with a thin, pliable, strong, almost invisible scar. Fibrin was laid in a thin layer across the wound, and epithelial tissue grew through it filling the gaps and sealing the wound. Scars, however, become thicker and more visible with age, though less pliable and strong. When we get older, we do not produce enough of the protein eating enzymes that control the amount of fibrin the body deposits into the wound. This leaves less space for the epithelial tissue to grow through. This over deposition or over expression of fibrin can be seen (and felt) in fibrocystic breast disease, uterine fibromas, postoperative scar tissue (especially in seniors after abdominal surgery), and in post injury contractures and fixations. Folks who produce too much fibrin get blood clots, deep vein thrombosis, and arteriosclerosis as fibrin is the matrix for all of these.[6]

Three. The enzymes are immuno-modulative. If the immune system is cranked up too high as in MS, Rheumatoid Arthritis, and Lupus, the enzymes tone the system down and then eat away at the CICs they're creating to attack their own tissue. If the system is down too low, the enzymes will boost production of the bodies natural killer cells, improve the action of the FC receptors of the white blood cells, and, overall, improve bug killing action.[7]

Four. And finally, the last major action of these enzymes is to keep the blood clean. As the carrier of oxygen and nutrients, our blood is the river of life. As the bearer of metabolic waste and necrotic derbies, the blood is also the river of garbage. In ideal worlds with perfectly healthy and strong individuals, the trash in the blood is supposed to be cleaned on its first pass through the liver. Since 99.9% of us over the age of one don't have clean livers, the cleansing action tends to get delayed. As the toxic load on the blood increases, so does its ability to flow smoothly, deliver oxygen, and decrease nutrients. Protein-eating enzymes aid the liver to out process this gunk and eat away at excess fibrin in the blood while decreasing platelet aggration. A nifty way to keep the blood thin, clean, and flowing.[8]

Most of us learned in physiology that old age begins at 27; this was Dr. Wolf's finding when he discovered that the human body's production of proteolytic enzymes begins to wane at that age and has a profound drop by 35. (Most of our aches and pains set in between 27 and 35; statistically our greatest drop in fitness, agility, and conditioning occurs between 27 and 35. In most, our looks change dramatically between 27 and 35. Think about it.)

In sports medicine enzymes will:

1 Keep micro injury from becoming macro injury.[9, 10]

2 Reduce inflammation.[11]

3 Speed healing.[12]

4 Prevent excesses of scar tissue or eat away at existing scar tissue.[6]

5 Improve blood rehology, especially in those athletes prone to severe dehydration or using EPO to increase red blood cell count. (In these athletes this drug causes the blood to get as thick as yogurt, yuck, greatly increasing the risk of blood clotting diseases.)[8]

6 Eliminate the need for the constant use of non-steroidal anti-inflammatory drugs (NSAIDs) and thereby prevent the major cause of visceral (internal organ) dysfunction, toxicity, and death in athletics. (After a particular New York marathon where a major US drug firm gave away samples of its over-the-counter ibuprofen, four runners died from the kidney failure that came from the combined result of dehydration and ibuprofen use.)

With over 160 peer-reviewed, mostly double-blind studies to verify their effectiveness, systemic enzymes are used by almost every Olympic team in Europe and most European pro sports teams. Currently many of the teams in the NFL, NHL, NBA, and Major League Baseball have discovered enzymes and are using them to keep their expensive players from being poisoned into retirement or death by the NSAID drugs.

During their heyday, the Eastern block nations were buying millions and millions of enzyme tablets through third parties in the West and secreting them behind the iron curtain. Not one got to a hospital or patient; the entire lot went to their sports training centers to prevent injury, speed workout recovery, and allow the eastern block athletes to maintain their impossible eight-hour a day training schedule without overtraining or incurring injury!

With that lead-in, you'll want to know which enzymes to use and how much! For maintenance, decreasing the wear and tear, and to avoid the use of NSAIDs, an athlete should take systemic enzymes, at least 5 tablets or capsules TID (three times a day) between meals. During injury states take the systemic enzymes 10 TID during the acute phase of injury (the first 72 hours), then reduce the dose to 5 TID. There is no LD 50 for enzymes; in other words, they are not toxic at any level of dosing.

After injury or surgery, we should be trying to restore as much, or more, of our prior ability. We'll go for more, and we'll do it faster if we put the nutritional needs of rehab on the same level of importance as the exercise we do.

Nutritional Needs

Now that we've covered the needs to rebuild tissue after hard training and play, we still have not spoken about the nutritional needs of the remainder of the body! After all, we don't just add gas to our car; we need oil, transmission fluid, brake fluid, coolant, and electricity! Even more goes into running our engine(s) than just the nutrients named above. Most high level athletes and health seekers dose themselves with 20 to 50 tablets and capsules of various nutrients each day in order to cover all of the nutritional bases and to ensure the chemistry is there for optimum performance. For those who have been at it long enough, just the sight of all those pills is enough to cause nausea. Plus, all of those tablets are very difficult to carry around if you're a traveling pro or college athlete. There are now all-inclusive powders on the market that contain all of the vitamins, minerals, and nutrient factors one needs for regular maintenance. (The demands of rehab would cause you to have to take some pills over and above the powder, but, overall, the number of supplements to eat or carry with you are greatly reduced.) These powders can be made into shakes; most of the companies even provide a handy closed-top shaker to take with you. These products can form the foundation for a superior athletic supplementation program.

So, now you have the nutritional wherewithal to both maintain your performance best and fix the glitches that inevitably come with having an active fitness lifestyle.

References

1. *Histology*, Arthur W. Ham. Lippincott Co., 1961 pg.209.

2. Ibid., Pg.267.

3. www.doctor-wallach.com/depletion.html

4. *Wall Street Journal*, 20 Apr. 1999.

5. *Enzymes – A Drug of the Future*, Prof. Heinrich Wrba MD and Otto Pecher MD. Published 1993 Eco Med.

6. Carrillo A., R.: *Clinical examination of an enzymatic anti-inflammatory agent in emergency surgery.* Arztl. Praxis 24 (1972), 2307.

7. Kunze R., Ransberger K., et at; *Humoral immunomodulatory capasity of proteases in immune complex decomposition and formation.* First International symposium on combination therapies, Washington, DC, 1991.

8. Ernst E., Matrai A.; *Oral Therapy with proteolytic enzymes for modifying blood rheology.* Klin Wschr. 65 (1987), 994.

9. Worschhauser S.; *Conservative therapy for sports injuries. Enzyme preparations for therapy and prophylaxis.* Allgemeinmedizin 19 (1990), 173.

10. Zuschlag J., M.; *Prophylaxis of soft tissue injuries in contact sports – enzyme preparations for the reduction of sports inabilities stemming from injuries.* Der Allgemeinarzt 16 (1991), 1285-1287.

11. Blonstein J., L.: *Oral enzyme tablets in the treatment of boxing injuries.* The Practitioner 198 (1967), 547.

12. Baumuller M., *The application of hydrolytic enzymes in the treatment of soft tissue distortions of the ankle.* Allgemeinmedizin 19 (1990), 178.

NOTES

Chapter 3
Tools for Recovering and Rebuilding
● ● ● ● ● ●

Before we actually get to learn about the different types of injuries, we need to learn what we can do to reduce the immediate effects of the injury, i.e., swelling, pain, and loss of function. Then we need to learn techniques to jump start the healing process without increasing inflammation (swelling and pain). And finally, we need to touch on rehabilitation techniques to restore full function, full strength, and pain-free full-range of motion to the affected area.

What happens to an area during an injury? Depending on the extent of the damage, you will have a degree of loss of function which may last for just a few minutes, in the case of a minor injury, to days or weeks, in the case of a serious hurt. Sometimes there may be serious injury without loss of function. A fracture of the forearm is a good example of this. The old wives' tale says that if you can move your fingers, a forearm is not fractured -- bull dookies! I've seen Coles fractures, a condition where both forearm bones are broken straight across and the patients are still capable of moving not only their fingers, but their wrists as well. So while we can expect some loss of function with most injuries, having function does not mean an injury is minor.

Next on the list of things that happen during an injury is inflammation. This condition is defined as swelling with pain and redness. The blood vessels in the injured area react to the insult by opening up and dumping a lot of fluid in the area to splint it up, and with the distention (ballooning up) of tissue comes pain. All this is nature's way of telling you to keep off the injured area until it heals. And back when we had no way of dealing with injuries, it was as good as nature could do to cope. Things healed slowly, if at all, back then. Anthropologists have found many human skeletons from the olden days with unfixed injuries. These days the inflammatory mechanism of an injury is seen as slowing down the healing process. Why? Do we know more than nature? No, but we can heal injuries better with intervention and treatment than if things were left to themselves!

The inflammation that swells an area after an injury also brings with it a load of calcium to deposit in the affected area. Our bodies do not know what has been injured, whether it has occurred to soft tissue or bone. Always opting for the worst case scenario, the body thinks bones have been fractured and so brings a great deal of calcium with the first load of body fluid. This calcium is useful only if there has been a fracture. If muscle, fascia, periosteum, tendons, cartilage, or ligaments have been injured, the calcium is useless and can create a new problem, one called myositis ossificans (MO). MO occurs when the calcium that has been deposited in an area during the initial phase of injury hardens into a large bone chip. Most examples of myositis ossificans can be found in the deltoid muscles of ex-football linemen. Those sometimes ping pong ball-sized lumps in the delts are prime examples of hardened MO. Sprinters often have this injury to the front of the thigh. MO limits range of motion and creates painful motion because the muscle or tendon must grate over the rough slab or barnacle of bone in order to move. This creates constant irritation and inflammation, which draws more calcium to the area and keeps making the MO worse! We won't get into how to get rid of MO without surgery in this book, but we will deal with avoiding its occurrence.

> **When dealing with the first 72 to 96 hours of an injury remember the acronym RICE.**
>
> - **R**est
> - **I**ce
> - **C**ompression
> - **E**levation

Though we may think they are self explanatory, let's go over each of these points in depth.

Rest. That's just what it says. No "walking it off," no "one more forced rep," no "one more for the gipper." No nothing. Get on your butt, unless that's the part that's been hurt, and REST.

Ice. The information concerning the beneficial effects of ice treatment of an injury has been around for nearly 40 years. I still find folks, even some old-time doctors who want to put heat on a fresh injury. (An injury is considered to be in its acute or fresh stage for the first 72 to 96 hours. If for whatever reason the injury is re-injured, then the count begins anew). If you put heat on a new injury, you will increase the swelling. This will not only up the pain and swelling, but the increased swelling will tear the injured tissue further apart increasing the severity of the injury. The swelling may also cause a dangerous thing called a compartment syndrome where the internal pressure from the swelling is so great that it can damage nerves acting as a tourniquet, cutting off the blood supply and causing tissue or an entire limb to die! While compartment syndromes happen mainly in the forearms and the legs, the excessive swelling that heat causes a new injury is unwanted as it dumps more calcium, greatly increases pain, and generally slows down the entire healing process.

When using cold therapy, it is always best to use real ice, preferably crushed and held in a small garbage bag, or two placed directly over the injury. The first two minutes will burn and sting, but things will get very numb very soon. If you use a synthetic cold pack, place a moist to wet towel over the affected area before the cold pack is put on. Why? Ice burn. Real ice will never cause frostbite because it never gets any colder than 32 degrees. (Ice massage is the initial treatment for frostbite!) Cold packs often get considerably colder than 32 degrees and can cause the skin to be burned as in a light frostbite. Leave the ice on for no longer than 15 to 20 minutes. The prolonged cold, instead of closing the blood vessels to minimize and reduce swelling, begins to open them, allowing swelling. Most of us have had the experience of our hands being prickly hot after a long snowball fight. At first cold closes the blood vessels. The body does not want to cool off its blood supply as this would reduce its operating temperature from the norm. In a reaction to prolonged exposure to cold, the body opens the outside blood vessels in the cold area and shunts warm blood from its central core, the abdomen in order to heat the area up. In the rehab phase of injury care, we will take advantage of this physiological trick but avoid it during the initial phase of injury.

Compression. During or after ice applications, the injured area should be wrapped in a compression bandage. Most folks wrap an "Ace" bandage altogether wrong. Here are a few tips to get things right: start the wrap at a point below the injury. Below means a point furthest away from the center of the body. For example, if a knee has been injured, begin to wrap the Ace about 5 inches below the knee and wrap the bandage up toward the thigh by taking only half of the stretch out of the bandage and overlapping each spiral over the one below by half the width of the bandage. Starting the compression below the injury and wrapping up (towards the torso) forces the swelling back up to the general circulation. Wrapping it the other way will force the swelling into an extremity where it can get stuck and permanently distend (stretch) skin and tissue.

For the more "modern" of us, there are neoprene rubber and elastic braces for almost every joint and area that can provide compression without the hassle of winding and coming unwound. Often these types of braces also have stiffeners and joints to assist the ligaments that may have been injured taking the pressure on the metal or plastic joints takes the pressure off the real joint. A note of caution here, unless you've been instructed by a doctor to keep the compression bandage or brace on at night, take it off during sleep. Your blood pressure (BP) goes down during sleep and the body fluids pool, but worse, if a compression bandage is left on while the BP is down, the body may not have enough blood pressure to get blood past the bandage or brace. This is bad, so just to be sure take all compression articles off during sleep.

Elevation. When ever possible have the injured area resting at an angle that will allow it to drain downhill; it's basic, but you'll be surprised how many prolong their injured state simply by failing to elevate the affected limb.

Other Things You Can Do

Healing / Drawing Ointments. When I was a young grad student, my head was in the clouds trying everything that could possibly work to reduce and rehab injury. One day I went to my naturopathic tutor, Dr. Charles W. Turner, and told "Doc" that I was using an old patent medicine on injuries that seemed to both reduce the bruising and discoloration along with the effusion and pain. (It works by drawing the black and blue to the surface where it dissipates back into the circulation.) The stuff looked like black melted crayon. Doc Turner turned to look at me and said that he didn't have any more to teach me, I had just found the secret of the world!

These nifty ointments have been around for over a hundred years. Their formulas are simple iodine in an ointment base with a touch of oil of wintergreen (methyl salisalate). The oil of wintergreen dilates the pores and allows the iodine to flow transdermally (across the skin) into the tissues. Concentrations of iodine in tissue will increase the local metabolism, dissipate black and blues, reduce swelling and pain, relax muscles, and generally speed healing. Iodine is what the thyroid gland needs to make the hormone Thyroxin. This hormone speeds things up.

When using a drawing ointment, apply a dab to the affected area; heavy applications are not necessary. Rub the ointment in until the color disappears. Use this over strains and sprains, on bruises and contusions, any swellings or sore points. The only problem with ointments is getting them! Even most old-time pharmacists think they've been long gone, but not so.

Systemic Enzymes. The same enzymes we learned about before as a benefit to healing, when taken in higher doses during the acute phase of an injury, greatly serve to reduce the inflammation and pain. Ten tablets three times a day are what is needed during the first 72 to 96 hours of injury. After that, back off to the recommended dose for active folks, five tablets two to three times a day.

Androstene Creams. Androstene is a precursor to testosterone. Creams are absorbed some 95% while oral administration of Androstene shows only a 5% absorption rate. The body takes this Androstene and turns in into its own testosterone. This is a wonderful supplement to speed healing of all bone and soft tissue injury.

During the Vietnam war, every wounded and injured trooper was given androgens (testosterone like substances) to help them recover faster. Though the work has been "denied" because of the stigma anabolic steroids now have due to their misuse in athletics, many old combat surgeons and front line doctors remember giving these drugs in their proper therapeutic doses (not using 5 to 20 times the normal dose as athletes and bodybuilders use) and having the wounded heal in record times. We can reproduce these healing times today without the side effects of using synthetic hormone drugs. Androstene is natural, it gives your body the tools it needs to make it's own testosterone. The only warning is for gals: Do not use this supplement if you are pregnant.

Doc Turner's Old Time Poultices

Dr. Charles W. Turner was the first black Naturopath, Chiropractor, and Osteopath. Studying all of these systems of medicine after his return from the First World War (and without the aid of a GI bill which did not come until after the Second World War), he compiled a mass of information on natural healing techniques which he applied in his 60+ years as a healer. One of his favorites was the Kosher Salt Poultice.

This remedy draws swelling from an area, as fluid moves from lower to higher saline concentrations, taking with it metabolic waste the cells may be holding. At the same time, in the opposite direction minerals are moving transdermally into the affected tissue. These minerals alkalinize the area (injured tissue due to its destruction and the holding of metabolic waste tends to be acidic and the higher the acidity, the slower the rate of healing). The salt also contributes mineral building blocks for tissue repair. Doc Turner proved that fluid had been transferred from the injury to the poultice by weighing the poultice before application and then again right afterward. It was heavier! This despite evaporation and cooling over the course of 20 minutes!

Use this treatment after the first 72 hours has past.

Kosher Salt Poultice Ingredients

- Use one of these heating pads:

    Hydrocolator heating pad large enough to cover the affected area, or

    Electric heating pad free of cuts or tears – able to withstand being wet. The pads of preference are specifically made for moist heat.

- One box of kosher salt
- A medium sized towel

Spread salt over half the towel and pour water no hotter than 105 degrees over the salt to create a kind of brine. Place the heating pad over this and fold the free side of the towel over it. Place the salt side of this poultice over the injury and hold at medium heat for 20 minutes. Once done, have ice cubes in a small plastic bag and dab over the area for 5 minutes. This creates localized vaso constriction and locks in the minerals and alkalization longer. If the ice is not done, all of the good stuff will be carried away quickly by the increased circulation.

For extremities, i.e. feet, hands, elbows, etc., water heated to no more than 105 degrees can be placed in a bucket to which is added from 1/2 cup to 1 cup of the salt. Again hold for 20 minutes, dab with ice for 5, and you're done.

Do this treatment daily.

Ice Massage

Here we use the trick of bringing blood from the inside / out instead of trying to force an increase of circulation from the outside / in. This method is useful for deep or thick areas. Heat applications used to stimulate circulation only penetrate into tissue some 1/2 to 1-1/2 inches. If, as in the case of a back, buttock, or thigh injury, the injured tissue is very deep, then no increase in circulation will be had at that level from superficial applications of heat. Remember that ice left on for over 20 minutes brings blood to an area from the inside / out. Now we'll see how to apply this.

> **Ice Massage Ingredients**
>
> • Cup full of ice cubes, or
> • Freeze water in a small paper cup

Take a cup full of ice cubes and gently rub the area with one ice cube, drawing small circles. When that cube is gone, use another. Do this procedure for 20 to 40 minuets. It may be more convenient to freeze water in a small paper cup. Peel the paper away and massage. As the ice melts, peel away more of the cup.

Do this 1 to 3 times a day.

We'll be making suggestions as to the use of these aids to recovery as we progress in our studies.

NOTES

NOTES

Chapter 4

Degrees of Injury - Goals for Recovery
• • • • • •

Usually this far in a sports medicine book for professionals, i.e., athletic trainers, exercise physiologists, physicians, etc., we get into the orthopedic tests done as a routine part of injury evaluation. However, this is a book for laymen, the absolute best advice I can give you is to see your doctor if:

The injury is bad.

You are knocked unconscious.

Something happens to an eye, tooth, testicle, penis, or breast.

You lose function in a limb for more than a couple of minutes.

You have radiating pain down the inside of the left arm.

You have radiating pain from the neck down an arm.

You have chest pain.

You have abdominal pain (increasing rigidity of the abdomen).

You suspect a fracture.

You don't remember your name, address, or other personal data.

You are cut or punctured.

You incur a blow to the head (any degree of concussion can kill).

You have fluid dripping from your ears after a blow to the head.

You have a swollen extremity.

You are hurt and scared.

You just plain don't know what you have.

Have someone take you to a doctor or emergency room immediately.

There are some 1,500,000 sports injuries needing medical attention each year! And don't think that just because the game is among children, they can't get seriously hurt! Yearly, in junior high school and high school football alone, there are some 15,000 injuries, 5000 of them serious enough to need surgery or to produce crippling disability. Nationwide, 25 to 30 kids die every year playing or practicing football.

You soccer moms out there thinking that you've spared your child the dangers of American football, think again. Shin fractures and compartment syndromes of the leg permanently damage hundreds of children playing soccer every year. Not to mention the brain damage, cervical nerve damage, and arthritis incurred from "heading" the ball. Heading the ball in soccer is about as smart as spearing is in football – with one exception. Spearing is illegal by rule and unethical for coaches to teach. The same is not true for heading in soccer!

Never, never, never neglect an injury. Sports may seem like combat but in all reality, it is far from it. The sacrifices we ask of our service personnel in wartime are not what we expect of kids and adults merely playing a sport. Sport is a game, not war. (You sideline coaching parents listen up.) Hurt your body and neglect it, and you will pay in the future with arthritis and dysfunction; that's a given. Enough preaching.

Once the injury has been evaluated and the degree of the damage diagnosed, we then have several options according to the degree of damage. However, all injuries need to be treated using the RICE protocol at first.

- **Rest**
- **Ice**
- **Compression**
- **Elevation**

First Degree Injuries

An athlete can play with first degree injuries if supportive taping or bracing is worn. Elastic braces and ace bandages do not constitute a SUPPORTIVE structure.

Athletic tape, or the material in the brace, has to make up for the laxity in injured ligaments. Therefore, they must restrict the range of motion in a joint to prevent further damage to tendons and ligaments. Don't depend on your doctor to tell you what bracing is best. Nine out of ten times he really does not know! If he is an orthopedist, he may send you to a brace maker. The school doctor should send an athlete to the athletic trainer for both rehab and taping of the area. Most ERs don't know what to recommend for a first degree injury that gives support and allows play. Seek out a pro on injury support during sports – a Certified Athletic Trainer.

Athletic Trainers are college-trained experts on the reduction, rehabilitation, and support of athletic injuries. There was a time when these experts were found only in colleges, but now high schools around the country have recognized the need to hire these caregivers. There are three professional organizations certifying the competence of athletic trainers. They are:

- American Athletic Trainers Association / American Sports Medicine Association
- The National Athletic Trainers Association
- The United States Sports Academy.

A certification from any of these organizations guarantees competence. Some states license Athletic Trainers, but with eastern states these licensers are more a sign of belonging to the "correct" political group and may not fully denote professional competence.

Second Degree Injuries

Second degree injuries are more serious, with more extensive damage to ligaments, tendons, and muscles. With this category of injury, several days or weeks must be taken to reduce the immediate effect of the injury and then restore function, strength, and range of motion. Do not play with a second-degree injury until your physician clears you! Further stress on the weakened and hurt part will make the injury more extensive and serious!

Third Degree Injury

A third degree injury is the worst kind. Here the player has a full tear of a muscle, tendon, or ligament. Here a spot where a tendon is attached to a bone may have pulled that bony piece clear off the shaft or joint platform. This is also where fractures and serious dislocations live. Third degree is where you don't want to be. Healing, casting, or surgery is not enough to recover from a third degree injury: a full bout of rehab and neuro muscular reeducation is needed to insure full function, strength, and range of motion after one of these injuries.

NOTES

NOTES

Chapter 5
Getting Fit To Play
● ● ● ● ● ●

Don't play to get into shape – get into shape to play. Many folks, doctors included, don't know the physiological difference between activity and conditioning. Activity is sport or play; it involves a skill and the fitness needed to perform that skill. Activity can also be damaging and tear down the body. Conditioning is exercise and the acquisition of the fitness needed to safely perform the sport. You don't get fit from doing a sport; you get fit for it!

Experience has shown us that specifically conditioned athletes have lower incidences of injury than non conditioned players and that when they do become injured, their injuries tend to be less severe than those of athletes in poor condition. The Navy Seals have a motto: *"train hard / fight easy,"* and this is how it should be. Conditioning exercise should specifically prepare an athlete by developing the strength, endurance, agility, and flexibility he or she will need to easily perform the skills demanded by the sport. The play itself should not be that much of an endeavor because the conditioning and skills training beforehand should have been harder than the game itself demands!

Each sport makes its own demands of the body, so the conditioning for one won't necessarily get you ready for another. A good example of this is seen in college when football players at the end of that season go into wrestling. Even though the football players have had an entire season of conditioning and play for football, it doesn't amount to a hill of beans when they get on the mat for the first wrestling practices and workouts. The football athletes are on the edge of the mat wheezing, puking, and trying to stop the muscle cramps just like the guys who had not worked out since last year!

Though there is definite "specificity" in conditioning, there are also certain power, agility, and endurance-producing exercises and practices that should be undertaken in all sports and by all athletes.

In the US we like to think of ourselves as being on the cutting edge, leaders in all endeavors, and ahead of the game in all things. This attitude may be true in most things, but it is definitely not true in sports medicine or athletic conditioning. Typically, America's ivory towers of sports medicine and exercise physiology are 20 to 30 years behind Scandinavia and Eastern Europe in theory and application. As an example, the top textbooks in exercise physiology on the development of strength and power are from Scandinavian physiologists. Romania's former national weightlifting coach was scoffed at by American academics when he described the training techniques he and the Communist Block in general utilized to build their gold medal powerhouse teams. They did not scoff for long. On trying out the techniques, mostly in an attempt to discredit the Eastern Block's methods, low and behold it turned out that they worked! The Romanian coach now heads up the US Olympic Weightlifting Team!

Most of the powerful Iron Curtain competitors were relatively small and poor countries. How could these nations with their small gene pools hope to compete against the powerhouses of genetic variety such as the US with its huge racial mix and the Soviet Union with its hundreds of nationalities. These large nations could custom fit a genetic type to a sport. The smaller countries had to work with what they had. What mix of things did the likes of Romania and East Germany do to produce athletes of such superior ability? The answers were threefold:

1 True Strength Training

2 Plyometric Power Training

3 Systemic Enzymes

True Strength Training

What do we mean by the term, True Strength Training? Strength is the ability to apply force. Most of what passes for strength training in the West today is simply modified bodybuilding, and as Russian strength coach Pavel Tsatsouline says, bodybuilding is the worst thing that ever happened to weight training. Bodybuilding works with moderate resistance with moderate numbers of repetitions, in very strict movement with the aim of producing muscular hypertrophy. Hypertrophy is defined as an increase in the size of an existing structure. Bodybuilders use techniques that balloon size without producing significant gains in strength or producing strength that is adaptable to sports performance. I'll explain how that works in a bit.

True strength training uses very heavy weights, few repetitions, and they do something unthinkable in bodybuilding - they cheat. In other words they use their whole body to help perform the lift. Like Bruce Lee's principle of putting the whole body mass behind a punch! This is not the recipe for safety in commercial gym settings where worries about injury liability outweigh performance physiology. Neither is it the recipe for a body builder's kissibly beautiful biceps. But whole body involvement is the recipe for functional strength. Skill movement in martial arts, sport, dance, or any activity involves the whole body, never one joint at a time. Training only one joint without synergistic involvement of the rest of the body produces strength that has little transference to real movement during performance. When involving the whole body, strength is amplified into power (strength over time). Proper strength training does not produce a lot of hypertrophy (bloating). Instead it produces a change in muscle known as hyperplasia where a muscle bundle splits and becomes two or more overlapping muscle bundles. The result is not the bloated, soft, easily lost size of the bodybuilder but plywood strong, dense muscles with lasting usable strength.

Here again we have one of the differences between European sports science and the Yanks – most physiologists here don't believe hyperplasia occurs in humans. In Europe hyperplasia has been a scientific given for 20 plus years, and they've adjusted their training methods accordingly with great success.

Notice the difference in size between bodybuilders and Olympic weight lifters. The smallest Olympic lifter is considerably stronger, pound for pound, than the biggest bodybuilder despite the size difference. Also, according to studies done at two separate Olympics, the weight lifters are also the second most flexible, balanced, and agile athletes there; the gymnasts are the first. Watch a bodybuilder move – flexibility, agility, and balance are definitely not strong points of their training or their being. Now, watch the balance of an Olympic lifter doing a clean and jerk; try the technique yourself if you don't think there's much to it! Then, watch that lifter get out from under a fully loaded barbell held over head! Strength, balance, and agility; they sound like traits needed in most sports, do they not? Next, feel the difference in the muscle. Show muscle feels doughy to a hard squeeze, like the muscles on a dystrophic child. Now squeeze the arm of an Olympic lifter or a power lifter. Solid steel covered by flesh. Show or performance? Posing or movement? Kata or Combat; for which shall you train? The physiological law of training specificity demands that one has to condition the muscles against the loads that the endeavor will demand from them. Bodybuilding is a non-contact sport getting you ready to pose and very little else. Strength training gets you ready to perform, to excel, and to strive.

Next the Communists had to develop an advanced way of turning the strength their techniques developed into power. Training slowly teaches you to move slowly. While slow performance is initially needed to learn the proper performance of a skill, practice must be sped up after learning to insure proper performance. Most sports demand explosive movements against resistance. That resistance can come either from gravity (as in gymnastics), a medium (such as water in swimming), or an opponent (as in judo or wrestling). Explosive movements against the weights can be done safely if proper training in its biomechanics is done beforehand. (This is definitely one not to try at home boys and girls, unless you've got the supervision of an exercise physiologist knowledgeable in the safety of such techniques.)

Mind you, I said Exercise Physiologist NOT personal trainer. What's the difference between the two? It's like the difference between someone who gets their black belt by attending two or three weekend seminars as opposed to someone who masters an art by spending years learning it's discipline in a temple. ('Nuff said).

Plyometric Power Training

Explosiveness against weights only partially builds the ability to produce power. To fill this need of sport, the Eastern Block exercise science folks developed Plyometric training. Here in the States some folks have fancied up some aspects of plyometric training with giant rubber balls and fancy equipment. You don't need any of those.

Let's first answer the basic question as to what plyometric exercise is. Plyometrics are exercises that involve an explosive movement of the extremities that propel the entire body. The wind-ups to these movements are usually full-body and the full body learns how to cooperate in producing great speed and explosiveness that transfers directly to a sport skill. One example of plyometric work you may have seen involves athletes zigzag-jumping over knee-high benches side to side. The most common plyometric exercise involves jumping up onto a bench some 20 to 25 inches high with both feet. Then the athlete jumps off to the rear and down again, absorbing the downward energy on the return, then uncoiling it to jump up once again. The Soviets trained all of their athletes, from the archers to the fencers to the shooters to the wrestlers in plyometrics. They found the balance, precision, anaerobic conditioning, and power developed by this work were useful for all athletes in all sports.

Plyometric Drills

Standing Jump

Start with a sturdy table or locker-room bench a little lower than kneecap high. Stand back away from the bench a distance less than arm's length. Windup by squatting down and swinging

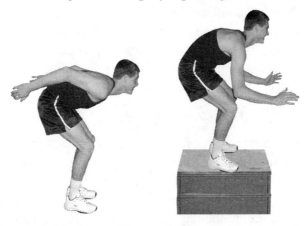

your arms behind you. Now swing your arms forward and leap up onto the bench. Reverse the squat and leap to get back down. As you land back on the floor, use the absorbing of the downward force to squat once again and windup for the next leap.

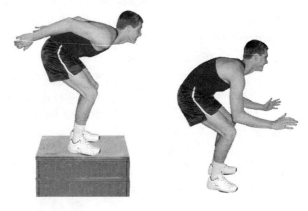

Start by doing 5 to 10 jumps for 3 to 4 sets. After you've attained a good level of balance and rhythm on the movement, go for time. Start at 30 seconds at first, then add 30 seconds more to each set. As you get stronger and faster, you should top off a set at two or three minutes. For example:

Week one: 4 sets of 5 reps.
Week two: 4 sets of 7 reps.
Week three: 4 sets of 10 reps.
Week four: 3 sets of 30 seconds.
Week five: 3 sets of 1 minute.
Week six: 3 sets of 1 1/2 minutes.
Week seven: 3 sets of 2 minutes.

Zig Zag Jumps

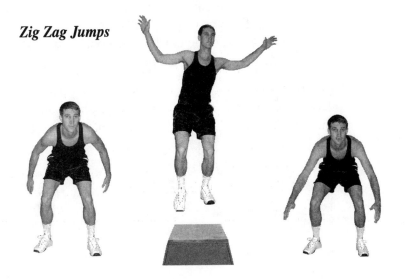

From the end of a low narrow bench, jump up and over the bench to land on the opposite side. Again use the force of landing to wind you up for the next jump. Plyometric work can also be done for the explosive muscles of the upper body.

Clapping Pushups

Basic. Get into the push up position with your feet wide apart for stability. You hands should be just outside of your shoulders with the thumbs pointed in the same direction as your head. This

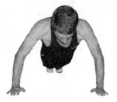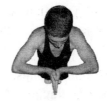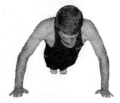

will take some pressure off the wrists and rotator cuff muscles of the shoulder. Push up explosively and while going up bring both hands together and clap. Do as many as you can for 3 sets. In the beginning, expect to crash to the floor a few times. This is normal, so do the exercise on a mat or thick carpeting.

Intermediate. After that, clapping your hands becomes relatively simple, so do the explosive push up and clap your hands on your chest. Again, do 3 sets of as many as you can perform.

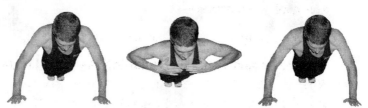

Advanced. There are two forms of the advanced clapping pushup. One has the person clap their hands together as many times as they can on each pushup; the other claps chest, then hands or chest, then hands repeatedly on each pushup. Doing these is not as hard as you might think.

My warning goes out to those athletes over 35 with OJS (Old Jock Syndrome). Your rotator cuff muscles either won't like you doing upper body plyometric work, or they simply won't let you. It's okay; you don't need that upper body speed anymore.

You're old enough that you should be able to play your team games for a few more years using more savvy and stealth than pure athletic ability. That's how life is; accept it. There is nothing sorrier than an aged thirty-something getting the crap beaten out of him under the boards by mere kids in a half court game! You should put more effort into playing individual games; the body lasts longer in those. Besides, as we get older we should be playing less and working out more. The first destroys the body; the second builds it.

A typical day for a Communist block athlete would go something like this:

Stretching. Not the slow static mamby-pamby passive stretching we advocate here but an active stretching that actually produces strength.

Progressive Resistance Training. Strength work at the afore–mentioned low reps, low sets, and high weights. For example, 3 sets of 3 to 5 repetitions with 80 to 95% of a 1 RM. An RM is the maximum weight you can move in that exercise for 1 repetition.

Plyometric Exercises

Skills Training. Practice in the actual sport.

Aerobic or Anaerobic Conditioning. As needed by the sport. What is anaerobic conditioning? Everyone can more or less describe aerobic exercise as working out the heart and lungs to develop endurance. This description would be correct, and we'll add one thing. In aerobic exercise, oxygen is the primary fuel the body uses to maintain its work load. You literally burn oxygen. Anaerobic exercise, on the other hand, does not involve long steady bouts of work but short and super intense rounds of exercise. In this type of work, oxygen is either not available to the muscles due to the intensity of muscular contractions which cut off blood supply, or the work bout overloads the body beyond its ability to deliver oxygen to all of the working parts. In this type of work, the cells burn glycogen or blood sugar as their primary fuel instead of oxygen.

Olympic free style wrestling is the best example of an anaerobic sport. Free style wrestlers are the best conditioned athletes, both aerobically and anaerobically, as the demands of their skill are so great. Conditioning for anaerobic ability involves nearly endless repetition of exercise drills involving one burst of energy after another. Athletes wind up breathless, nauseous, dizzy, and the number of precious-energy producing centers of the cells known as mitochondria just build and build. This increases both the stores of potential energy as well as the actual furnaces to burn that energy in the cells. The result—longer, stronger, more controlled and able bursts of skill performance.

The third secret is not a training method but a physiological realization as to three drawbacks of intense training. Inflammation, micro injury, and immune system depression. These are the main limiting factors on sports performance.

All conditioning and skills training produces inflammation. Muscles, tendons, ligaments, bursa, periosteum all react to hard training by swelling and becoming painful. The more this accrues, the less intensely the athlete will participate in the training. Micro injuries occur every day in skill and conditioning exercise. These tiny injuries are not enough to sideline an athlete, but they accumulate and, sooner rather than later become a macro injury demanding rest. Over and above the lapse in training, both micro and macro injuries produce scar tissue (fibrosis) which limits the range of motion in the limb and creates the potential for further injury.

The one aspect unrecognized until the 60s was that intense training schedules lowered the body's immunity. Every day of hard training is followed by two to three days of immune system suppression. When an athlete tags too many days of training together without adequate rest, the immune system goes into steep decline, sometimes to the point in some athletes, such as marathoners, where it dies out all together. There is now even a professional journal for immunology issues in sports medicine. What armament did the Iron Curtain countries use to combat these three deadly foes to performance?

Through the 40s and into the 60s, Cortico Steroid drugs were used against the inflammation. These drugs had nasty side effects such as water weight gain, death of bursa (the tissues that lubricate the articulation of muscle to bone), weakening the tendons, osteoporosis, extreme mood swings, and more. None of those are conducive to high level athletic performance! They had no answers for the issues of fibrosis and immune system depression. Then came the late 60s and everything changed.

In the constant search for substances to improve performance, the East Germans took notice of a preparation that was gaining favor on the other side of Germany – Human Growth Hormone or HGH.

This product was used by physicians to naturally reduce inflammation, eat away at fibrosis, and modulate immune function.[1] Its components were already approved for use in boxing to reduce brain swelling due to practice or matches.[2] When the product was tested, it surpassed all expectations as an inflammation controller. What's more, it kept micro injuries from becoming macro injuries and ate away at the limiting fibrosis of older injuries.[3] When an athlete was injured, use of the product caused that athlete to heal faster than ever before.

Use of cortico steroids could be dropped.   When the International Olympic Committee (IOC) banned cortico steroid use in 1975, most of the Eastern Block countries did not even blink. Their athletes were already off the anti-inflammatory drugs and performing harder, healing faster, staying healthier, and maintaining their ranges of motion all through the use of the those same enzymes.

There will be some who'll scoff and say that all of the Eastern Block's sports' greatness came through the use of anabolic steroids. Not so! Our athletes used the same dope and used as much as the reds did! So why were the Communist kids that much better? (The one place where Soviet and East German drug science did excel was in covering up drug use.) The Olympic athletes themselves called the Olympics in Atlanta the Human Growth Hormone Games. HGH is the favored drug of

Olympians since there is presently no test to determine its use. But HGH has some horrid side effects on healthy young people; so bad, in fact, they make anabolic steroids look good. But that's a story for another time.

The IOC seems impotent to stop drug use because spectators come to see records shattered. Without drugs, such sports as cycling, speed skating, and track and field would be boring events where this year's times and distances would be no better than the last games, and those not much better than they were in the '64 and '68 games! The result would be a drop-off in viewers and a drop-off in sponsorship. The bribing scandal concerning the Utah winter Olympics did more than anything else to show that the Olympics were no longer about the glory of amateur sport; they're all about the glory of money for the promoters, the hosts, and the potential winners. In this vein, the IOC has nothing to learn from the WWF about the link between money, promotion, and performance; the IOC wrote the book!

If you are into extreme performance, if you are into real training – overdoing and pushing the envelope of human performance – then take heed of what they did behind the Berlin wall. The Comrades got it right! Now 30 years later we need to catch on. 'Nuff said.

References

1. Muller-Hepburn W.: *Anwendung von Enzymen in der Sportsmedizin.* Forum d. Prakt. Artes 18 (1970).

2. Bronstein J.L.: *Oral Enzyme Tablets in the Treatment of Boxing Injuries.* The Practitioner 198 (1967), 547.

3. Baumuller M. *Therapy of Ankle Joint Distortions with Hydrolytic Enzymes - Results from a double blind clinical trial.* In: G.P.H. Hermans, W.L. Mostred (eds.) Sports, Medicine and Health. Excerpta Medica, Amsterdam, New York, Oxford (1990), 1137.

NOTES

NOTES

NOTES

Chapter 6
Avoiding Excessive Exercise
●●●●●●

Now that the over-exercise craze of the 80s and 90s has passed, we know that excessive activity (such as marathoning and triathaloning) and excessive exercising (such as aerobic dance and 6-7 day a week lifting) can and does create disease states in the human body.

Many of the marathoners who claimed to be running from heart disease wound up dead from that very condition. The cause was not from genetic predisposition, as many of the running faddists have claimed, but from vascular scarring and inflammation caused by the volume of running they did. Some lifters, supplementing their training with high dosages of creatine, an over-the-counter supplement that bloats muscle up in size, wound up dead or nearly dead from muscle wasting and kidney failure. It seems that excessive creatine combined with dehydration creates a deadly condition known as Rhabdomyolysis. Those who survived the rapid muscle death did so only after extensive surgery removed the dead and dying tissue these lifters worked so hard to build! In other cases of overdoing, the immune systems of endurance athletes died, leaving them at the mercy of any old infection. One famous marathon runner got an infectious disease from his cat! Once the immune system is gone, it's gone forever. Most of the overdoers of the 80s and 90s are now nearly crippled from the excessive joint wear their activities caused. The overdoers of the late 70s are dead or in wheelchairs!

There is a guiding principle here: anything overdone hurts the body! From eating to exercise, that which is good can also be bad. Let's list the things that over-activity / over exercise can cause:

- Heart disease
- Decreased Immunity
- Kidney damage or failure[1]
- Excessive joint wear leading to crippling arthritis
- Adrenal gland dysfunction or failure (Addison's Disease)

With the kidneys and the adrenal gland, failure equals death.

Don't think that you're a special case, immune to these conditions because God gave you some special dispensation or strength he did not give the other folks who play your game! As good as you may be, *YOU ARE NOT SPECIAL.* Olympic gold medalists have developed these conditions. Many American and professional athletes have succumb to these conditions – why can't you? Train hard, play hard, then rest long. Remember that for every day of hard training or hard play there are 2 to 3 days of immune suppression to follow.

As general rules of thumb, those 27 and under need 2 days of complete rest in the week. That means no training or sports play of any kind during the rest days. Those over 27 need 3 days of rest. Over 40, 4 days of rest in the week. Violate these rules at your own peril. Remember – when it comes to immune system failure, adrenal failure, cardio vascular damage, or injury, the mantra is: *I AM NOT SPECIAL.* You overdoers can repeat the chant day and night over and over until it sticks in whatever gray matter your overtraining has left you.

References

1. MacSearraigh, E.T. M., Kallmeyer, J.C., Schiff, H.B.: *Acute renal failure in marathon runners*. Nephron 24:236-240. 1979.

NOTES

Chapter 7
Foot, Ankle, and Leg Injuries
● ● ● ● ● ●

By far the most common injuries in sports are those of the ankle, knee, and shoulder; all other injuries are also-rans in comparison to these major three. Moving in order of frequency we'll look at ankle injuries, the mechanisms by which they become hurt, and, as in each of these chapters, we'll go over how to reduce the injury, shield it from further insult, and completely and wholistically heal it, returning to our stated goal of full function, strength, and range of motion.

The ankle, foot, and leg are so interconnected that we cannot speak of injuries to one without covering injuries to the other. (Please remember that in anatomy the leg is everything from the ankle to the knee; it does not include the thigh.) At the ends of the muscles, attaching the muscles to bones, are the tendons. Tendons in that area go over both joints and end either just below the knee or just above it. Ligaments that hold bone to bone are numerous at the ankle and foot. Usually, while a twist or a pull may injure mainly one ligament, you can be sure that other ones were hurt in the injury as well. The actions many think of as being part of the ankle are actually those of the foot, and we will see how they interact.

But first we need a bit of an anatomy lesson. The ankle joint is made up of three bones:

1 The distal

2 The fibula

3 The tibia

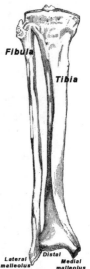

The distal (lower bone) connects the ends of the fibula and the tibia (the two leg bones). The ends of these two bones are called malleoli and the two form a mortise into which a bone called the talus of the foot fits. It is this joint (articulation) that allows the foot to move in flexion (toes towards your knee) and extension (toes away from your knee).

Below the ankle articulation we have the foot joint comprised of 7 small bones which give great movement potential and

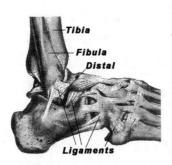

flexibility to the foot. It is at this joint that we can see the difference between inversion of the ankle (inner malleolus towards the midline of the body) and eversion of the ankle (outside malleolus away from the body's midline). (Just to confuse matters, it just so happens that eversion of the ankle produces inversion of the foot and inversion of the ankle produces eversion of the foot! Got that? OK!) So again flexion and extension occur at the ankle while inversion and eversion occur at the foot. Circumduction, a circular movement which draws a cone, is performed by using both the ankle and foot joints. In most all movements in sports and daily life, the ankle and foot joints are smoothly working together to produce the desired motion or stability.

Ligaments, the most important of which are at the ankle, hold the bones together. On the outside we have the Anterior Talofibular while the Anterior Tibiofibular Ligaments are in the front. In the rear, the Calcanialfibular ligament holds those bones together. On the inside of the ankle, we find quite a different arrangement with just one major ligament, the Deltoid – or three-headed ligament. This one spans from the front inside to the rear inside and holds the bones together while allowing for greater movement.

Next, tendons transfer muscle contractions to connecting bones to produce movement. At the outside of the ankle and foot there are the 3 peronial tendons. These tendons pull the foot to the outside (ankle inversion) and help to do push off motions with the

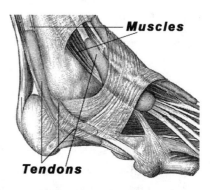

Muscles

Tendons

foot. At the front, we have the Anterior Tibialis muscle and tendon which pull the toes and foot up toward the knee. Also, here are the tendons of the muscles which not only pull your toes up off of the floor but also help to pull the entire fore-foot up.

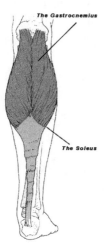

The Gastrocnemius

The Soleus

To the inside of the ankle are the tendons from the muscles that dig the toes into the floor. These structures also help to point the foot away from the knee. At the rear of the ankle, we have an interesting arrangement – three muscles come into a common tendon, the Achilles. These muscles are:

- The Gastrocnemius
- The Soleus
- The Plantaris

They are used to push the foot off of surfaces by pointing it. Underneath the Achilles is the Posterior Tibalis muscle and tendon which not only help in pushing off but also turn the foot inward (eversion of the ankle). All of these muscles attach just below the knee while the grastocnimius attaches above the knee at the lower rear end of the thighbone.

The bulk of ankle injuries involve turning the ankle out and the foot in. These are known as eversion injuries. Swelling will occur and, depending on the degree of the injury, the ligament may be:

- **First Degree**. Partially torn in a minor way
- **Second Degree**. Torn part way through
- **Third Degree**. A full tear

At times the ligament is so strong that instead of a third degree tear, the ligament will come off of the bone, by ripping a chunk of bone with it when it is forced to stretch. This is known as an avulsion. **Avulsions** are treated as fractures and heal faster, and with less fuss, than a third degree ligament tear which must be repaired surgically.

All injuries produce some loss of function and strength. How long this lasts depends on the extent (degree) of the injury. Lack of use can last for anywhere from a minute or two to days or weeks. This is the reason why all injuries need to be evaluated by personnel qualified to determine the extent of the injury. (Coaches anxious to win games don't count here. Only certified sports medicine personnel such as certified athletic trainers and orthopedic physicians.) An athlete with a first degree injury can be taped or braced and return to the game after a short period of ice treatment. Such is not the case with the other two degrees. Attempting to play with a serious injury (second or third) will result in that injury becoming worse and possibly causing further injury. Other joints will attempt to compensate for the weakness and reduced function of the injured area.

The school year injunction to "walk it off" is as stupid as trying to walk off getting hit by a car! Just as stupid is the "old coaches tale" that "if you can move, it isn't fractured." Unless you're a trooper in the field in times of war, the only thing to do when you or someone else is injured is to do "RICE" and get medical attention. Unlike war, sports involves games and are not worth causing permanent or crippling injury. There are tens of thousands of men, women, boys, and girls who awaken in the morning to the pains of sports-caused arthritis. This pain and its dysfunction follows them throughout their day, interfering with their daily activities, getting worse as the years pile on.

Most of this pain and degeneration could have been avoided if the athlete had pulled from play at the first sign of injury. Coaches, parents, and teams expect a level of sacrifice and suffering from the young that should only be asked for in times of dire need, such as war. It's just a game; get that through your, and everyone else's, head. No game, no matter how seemingly important it may be now, is worth the life-long pain and dysfunction that playing with an injury can cause. Okay, I'll get off of my soapbox now.

Whenever you have an injury to the ligaments, you also have an injury to the tendons that cross those ligaments! Injuries are never just localized to one anatomical structure. So an eversion sprain to the ligaments at the outside of the ankle will produce a strain to the tendons that lie over it. So most of the time when you have a sprain, you'll also have a strain. But it does not work the other way around! It is possible to strain a muscle where there are no joints underneath or stretch a tendon and not injure the ligaments of the joint that it crosses. (Just another example of how complex the human body is.)

Most Common Injuries

Eversion of the Ankle

This twisting out at the ankle and in at the foot causes a serious stretch (sprain) at the anterior Talofibular ligaments and the anterior Tibiofibular ligaments.   At times the athlete tries to counter the outward sway of the ankle by inverting strongly, usually causing another sprain to the Deltoid ligament.

With this injury, strains most often occur at the 3 Peronial tendons, especially the longus at the rear of the lateral (outer) malleolus. This tendon has the tendency to break free of the connective tissue which holds it in its notch resulting in the tendon clicking painfully out and over the posterior part of the malleolus and back in again. Many a football running back and wide receiver's career has been brought to an end by these thin tendons.

What to do to recover:

- RICE
- Treatment for strain
- Treatment for sprain
- Brace or tape, to get back into activity
- Active rehabilitation with weights - once cleared

Fibular Fractures

These can happen anywhere along the shaft or at the malleolus. Kicks, twists, and hard landings are the most usual causes. If there is an external force, like another player's foot, or if the body position is just right, leaning most of the weight of the athlete over the twisting ankle, the bottom (distal) end of the Fibula bone might fracture. With the popularity of skateboarding and in line-skating, these injuries are showing up more, not as simple fractures, but as Tri-Plane fractures. In other words, there are three breaks on two different bones, the fibula and tibia, going in 3 different planes or directions. Very

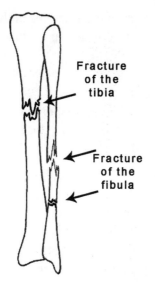

Fracture
of the
tibia

Fracture
of the
fibula

often these cannot be reduced by external manipulation and must be repaired surgically.

What to do to recover:

- Get medical attention
- Treatment for fracture
- Active rehabilitation with weights once cleared

Fallen Arches / Shin Splints

The two go hand-in-hand. At the bottom of the foot, attach the supportive musculature to allow movement of the foot while

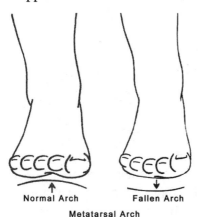

Normal Arch   Fallen Arch
Metatarsal Arch

holding the arch up. These attach at the other end on the front and sides of the shin. Downward pounding, as in running or gymnastics landings, causes the arch to drop, spraining the ligaments at the arch and causing the attached tendons and muscles to stretch. These then begin to tear off from the top end, resulting in shin splints.

Another cause of shin splints is the same pounding force that separates the two malleoli from each other. Between the fibula and tibia bones is a thin membrane connecting both called the Inter Osseous Membrane. This plastic-wrap-like sheet holds all of the blood vessels that feed the inside of the leg. The separation causes a tear in the membrane – OUCH!

A third cause of shin splints is stress micro fractures of the tibia, usually from running on hard surfaces with shoes that do not absorb shock well.

What to do to recover:

- Raise the arches in the shoes via arch supports or orthotics
- Get shoes with greater degree of heel cushioning
- Tape support for the foot
- Treatment for sprain
- Tape the leg to prevent bone spread

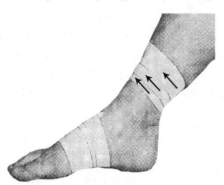

If all this plus rest (i.e., no running for 6 to 8 weeks) fails to resolve the shin splint, then go to the orthopedist and have the tibia x-rayed to check for stress fractures. Cast the leg for micro fractures.

Shin splint strapping

Compartment Syndromes of the Leg

In these injuries, an external force, usually a kick, causes a hemorrhage inside one of the three envelopes that form the inside of the leg. Pressure builds within the envelope, cutting off fresh blood circulation. If this pressure is not relieved by draining the blood, then death of the tissue from lack fresh blood supply will occur possibly leading to the need for amputation. ANY painful swelling of the shin or sides of the leg needs to be seen by a doctor "pronto." Draining the hemorrhage takes just a few minutes, though it can be quite dramatic. Soccer moms listen up! Aside from the head injuries and fractures in the sport, this is one of the most common injuries your kids will face.

What to do to recover:

- Get medical attention fast
- RICE afterwards
- Treatment for contusion / hemorrhage
- Recondition with weights

Tibial Fractures

The tibia is the longest and strongest bone of the leg, yet it can and does often break. In children, fractures can occur at the growth plate, just under the knee at what is known as the tibial plateau. Fractures at the shaft of the bone can also be caused by kicks or running into obstacles. Often times with tibial fractures a good deal of soft tissue is damaged, and if it is a compound fracture a good bit of blood might be lost. These factors all have to be taken into account when formulating a recovery program.

What to do to recover:

- Get medical attention
- Treatment for fracture
- Treatment for hemorrhage
- Treatment for strain
- Recondition with weights before attempting play!

Foot Bone Dislocations and Subluxations (Partial Dislocations.)

These are more common than one would think and are often misdiagnosed as plantar fasciitis. The seven bones of the rear foot can and do rotate out of position, causing sharp pain and dysfunction. Here someone expert in extremity adjusting must be consulted to put the bones back in place. Some podiatrists and some chiropractors know these adjustments. Not all of these doctors know how to adjust the foot, so ask before going to see them.

What to do to recover:

- Seek a chiropractor or podiatrists expert in extremity adjusting
- RICE
- Treatment for sprain
- Arch supports

Fractures of the Foot

Usually happens when an injured foot is stepped on.

What to do to recover:

- Get medical attention
- RICE (if no cast is applied)
- Treatment for fracture
- Supportive bracing and arch supports to return to play

Plantar Fasciitis and Heel Spurs

There is a membrane made of connective tissue (fascia) that resembles a weave of very fine white hairs. During most activities, this supporting membrane stretches and gives to meet the forces that are taken up by the foot. When it can't stretch any more, or if repeated injury has built up scar tissue within the fascia, the tissue will tear and attempt to rip itself from its connections at the forefoot and heel. The body will then react by drawing calcium to the area and cement the fascia to the bone and bingo, you've got a spur. Micro current electrotherapy and soft tissue manipulation such as Myo Fascial Release work best to relieve the pressure and pain, and to restore functionality to the foot. Nutrition and self-care must also be done to hasten the recovery and prevent its return.

What to do to recover:

- Soft tissue manipulation

- Micro current electrotherapy
- Treatment for bone spurs and arthritis
- Wear arch supports or orthotics daily especially when playing or practicing

Dislocated or Subluxed Fibula Heads

This is an injury most Orthopedists think they've never heard of or seen. It is often misdiagnosed as a Fibular Collateral Ligament Sprain of the Knee. The problem is the knee joint, and that ligament is some two inches above the site of pain. If the surgeon would just look a little south of the collateral ligament and notice that the head of the fibula is not where it should be, especially when compared to the non injured knee, things might get settled.

I've observed experienced physicians evaluate this injury and miss the diagnosis. When I pointed out the obvious deformity caused by the dislocation of the top of the fibula bone, something their "trained eye" missed, all I got was a huff. They had never been taught in school that the top of that bone could become dislocated or subluxed (partially dislocated). When I gently popped the dislocation back in and the patient's pain was relieved, returning the limb to full functioning, the doctors became believers! When I taught orthopedics, I always made sure the students knew about the condition, how to evaluate it, how to differentiate it from a knee injury, and how to reduce it.

What to do to recover:

- Find an MD, DO, ND, or DC who knows how to do extremity adjusting
- Treatment for sprain
- Tape or brace fibula head before activity to prevent recurrence (If you've dislocated this bone once, chances are it will happen again occasionally.)

Achilles Tendon Strain

This is the tendon that connects the 3 muscles of the calf at the rear of the leg to a common tendon. Here the Gastroc, Soleus, and Plantaris come together and attach to the heel bone (calcaneus). These muscles make it possible to point the foot towards the ground (plantar flex). Pushing off endeavors, as in sprinting or jumping, often tax this tendon.

In evaluating a strain of the achilles, the doctor or athletic trainer must palpate (feel) the outside edges of the structure and check for divots and fraying. If divots are found at the edges, the evaluator must then feel to see if there is troth between the divots. This indentation across the tendon indicates that the tendon is tearing along that line. If such continues, the entire tendon will rip apart creating a condition needing surgical repair.

What to do to recover:

- Get medical attention
- RICE
- Treatment for sprain
- When medically cleared, strengthen the tendon with weights and stretch for flexibility

Rehab For Foot, Ankle and Leg Injuries

Towel Gathering for Foot Injuries

Place a medium sized towel on a bare floor and sit in a chair at one end of it. Using only your toes pull the towel toward you

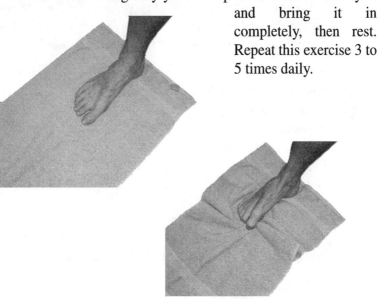

and bring it in completely, then rest. Repeat this exercise 3 to 5 times daily.

Calf Raises

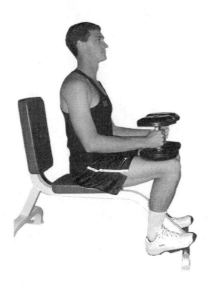

Using a leg press, standing calf, or seated calf machine, place your toes on the bottom edge of the footrest. Let your heels sink down as deeply as they can stretch, then raise the heels up as high as you can. The straight leg calf raise works the diamond shaped Gastroc muscle while the seated version is better for the Soleus muscle beneath the Gastroc and the smaller muscles of the ankle and foot. Since in most ankle injuries it is the smaller muscles that are most hurt, I prefer to use the seated version of the exercise with patients. Do 3 sets of 5 to 7 repetitions.

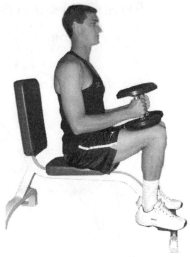

Foot Pull-ups

Tie a strong string, a bootlace, (in this case, a strap), to a 5 to 10 pound barbell plate. Hanging the plate on or beneath the foot on the injured side, tie the bootlace to the bottom of the laces on the

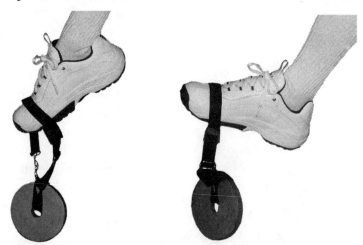

shoe you are wearing (in this case the strap is hanging from the front of the foot). Sit on a tall table or counter. Start from a toes toward the floor position and pull the foot up toward the ceiling.

Do as many reps as it takes to make the front of the shins burn. Rest about 2 minutes and try again. Do 3 sets this way. This exercise will strengthen the muscles at the front of the leg.

Calf Stretches

Stand on the edge of a stair step with only the balls of your feet, allowing the heels to hang off. Now sink the heels down as low as pain will allow. Remember take a stretch only to the first

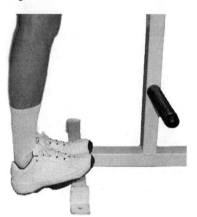

point of pain, then hold it there. As you progress, that first point of pain will occur further and further into the stretch. Hold for a slow count to twenty. Repeat 3 times.

NOTES

NOTES

_____

_____

_____

_____

_____

_____

_____

_____

_____

_____

_____

_____

_____

_____

_____

_____

_____

_____

_____

_____

_____

_____

_____

_____

_____

_____

_____

_____

_____

_____

NOTES

Chapter 8
Knee and Thigh Injuries
••••••

After ankles, the knee is the most injured joint in sports, dance, and exercise. Knees are among the most shallow and freely movable joints in the body. That freedom to move and change direction comes with a price, instability. The rule is that the deeper the socket and the more bone surrounding a joint, the more stable and less prone to injury it is.

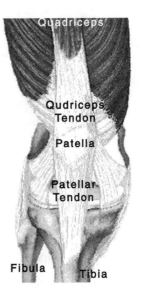

With knees we have a very shallow socket at the tibia allowing the ball found at the thighbone (femur) to glide in an ark up to 135 degrees and allow for rotation as well. To permit all this movement, the ligaments' structure of the knee is flimsy. There are two ligaments at the sides of the knee to hold things together from side to side, and two ligaments crisscrossing inside the knee to keep you from putting your foot in your mouth or losing your leg behind you when you step. At the front we have a ligament combined with a tendon from the bottom of the kneecap (patella) to its attachment at the tibial tuberosity below, and there is a tiny ligament in the back, at the hollow of the knee, to hold the cartilage found inside the knee in place. This cartilage, or menisci, are comprised of two semi-lunar pieces of a tough material that resembles a fibrous but smooth outer shell over an inner filling of mucous liquid. Its purpose is to deepen the joint, prevent bone to bone contact, and act as a hydrostatic shock absorber.

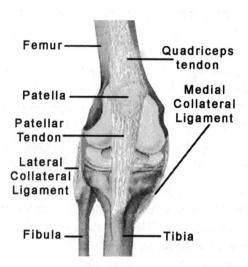

Femur

Quadriceps tendon

Patella

Medial Collateral Ligament

Patellar Tendon

Lateral Collateral Ligament

Fibula

Tibia

Think of the knee as a giant hinge. Movement for the hinge is provided by 4 sets of muscles. The large quadriceps in the front both bend (flex) the hip joint and straighten (extend) the knee. As the Quad prefix suggests, this muscle is made up of four heads or segments. The largest is the Rectus Femoris, then the Vastus Latteralis at the lower outside, and the Vastus Medialis at the lower inside. These 3 extend the knee to just shy of locking out. Taking the knee the last 15 to 20 degrees into its locked position is the tiny Vastus Intra Medialis. They are helped in the front by the longest muscle in the body–the Sartorius (or tailor's) muscle. While the quadriceps merely extend the knee, the sartorius extends and causes the lower extremity to rotate away from the body's midline (outward rotation.)

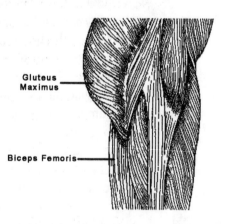

Gluteus Maximus

Biceps Femoris

Behind the femur we find the hamstrings; from outside to inside they are the Semi-Membranous, Semi-Tendonosis, and Biceps Femoris. These muscles, together with the Gastroc from the leg below, are in charge of bending (flexing) the knee. At their top end the Hamstrings also help the Gluteal muscles straighten (extend) the hip.

At the inside of the thigh there are the strong groin muscles (Femoral Adductors). These run from the "sit" bones of the pelvis to attach on the inner surfaces of the femur from midway down its shaft to just below the knee. These structures have the job of pulling the thigh in toward the body's midline. On the outside of the thigh connected to the top of the pelvis are the Hip Abductor muscles. Some of these muscles go to the just below the hip, and one to just below the knee. Though they are on the thigh, we'll deal with the Hip Abductors in the next chapter.

The bulk of knee injuries occur from a combination of forcible extension and torsion, in other words, straightening and rotating the knee at the same time while under some force (running, cutting, or someone falling on the limb).

Most Common Injuries

Sprain of the Collateral Ligaments

A sudden torque, a foot firmly planted while attempting to change direction during running, a kick against the side of the knee, all of these can cause the most common of all knee injuries. Of the two collateral ligaments, the inner (medial) is the one most often injured since exterior forces are more likely to land against the outside of the knee than against the inside. This force applied to the outside causes the joint to open on the inside forcing a stretching and tearing of the ligament.

What to do to recover:

- Get medical evaluation
- RICE
- Treatment for strain
- Treatment for contusion if strain received from outside hit
- Weights and stretching to restore strength, range of motion

Meniscus Tears

The menisci are connected to the tibial plateau by a ring ligament. The inner one is also connected to the medial collateral ligament so it can be pulled gently out of the way of the prominence at the center of the joint during rotational movement. If an injury to that ligament is bad enough, it will cause the meniscus to tear from that attachment, allowing the meniscus to float around the joint and possibly locking it up by jamming itself between the cruciate ligaments and the middle prominence of the tibia. OUCCH in spades!! This is called a bucket handle tear.

In some sports, heavy force is sufficient not only to cause a tear of that meniscus but of the outer one as well – the annular ligament. Though not as common as the medial meniscus tear, these are seen in serious knee injuries.

What to do to recover:

- Get medical evaluation
- RICE
- Treatment for sprain
- Treatment for contusion
- After a period of immobilization, stretch and do weights to restore range of motion and strength

Cruciate Ligament Tears

These are quite common in sports but most always occur in conjunction with other tears. For instance, the condition known as the unhappy triad of the knee is comprised of a sprained medial collateral ligament, a torn medial meniscus and an anterior curciate ligament tear. Of the two cruciates, the Anterior is the one most frequently injured as most blows or shocks to the knee come from the front and outside. To injure the posterior cruciate, the traumatic force would most likely have to have come from the rear.

What to do to recover:

- Get medical evaluation

- RICE

- In severe tears, surgical repair may be needed to insure stability (usability) in the joint. Hold off surgery until you've first tried to rehabilitate the joint. Orthopedists are first and foremost surgeons and many times will rush their patients into cutting. The old joke in sports medicine is that if you do nothing but rehab, your knee may hurt and lock out for some two years; if you do surgery, your knee may hurt and lock out for some two years!

- Treatment for sprain

- Treatment for contusion

- Restore range of motion and full strength with stretching and weights

Joint Mice

Frequently injuries fracture parts of the smooth cartilage within the joint causing a piece of it to come loose and float around. Also, semi-torn pieces of injured cruciate ligaments can flap around. Both of these can get into the space in the middle of the joint where the tibial prominence is and jam the joint, preventing either extension or flexion. There are manipulation techniques to unlock the joint and return almost immediately to full weight bearing, but after a locking event, a session of RICE should be done. With time (one to two years) the body will reabsorb floating segments of cartilage, but torn curates will continue to be a bother. If locking is excessive in occurrence then surgery might be considered to remove or repair the offending piece.

What to do to recover:

- RICE
- Treatment For sprain
- If joint won't unlock, seek a Chiropractor, Naturopath or Osteopath who knows how to adjust extremities

Patella Bursitis

Bursitis is an inflammatory condition of the sacs that produce the lubrication to smooth the movement of muscles and tendons over bones. With overuse or straining the tendons that run over them, the bursae tend to swell as a defensive reaction. This swelling can recur for years, whenever the joint is stressed. There are 13 bursa sacs around the kneecap (patella) and at times only the ones surrounding the kneecap from above swell (supra patella bursitis); sometimes only the ones surrounding the patella from below swell (infra patella bursitis). In more serious cases of bursitis, all of the sacs will swell. When this happens, you won't be able to really make out the kneecap or the tendon below it, and the knee joint area may look as large as the thigh.

What to do to recover:

- Treatment for inflammation
- RICE
- Do not train until inflammation is significantly reduced and mostly pain free movement is restored

Patella Tendonitis

In this condition the tendon / ligament combination that connects the bottom of the kneecap to the tibia is inflamed from having strained it. This structure is one of the only areas of the body where a tendon and a ligament are found together in one unit. This condition is rarely found alone and most always occurs with a protective infra patella bursitis.

Severe strains of this tendon may cause fraying at the edges that tear their way inward as the tendon / ligament fibers give. Most of these strains are minor, though painful and limit ability. Loss of range of motion and strength, high pain levels, and a lot of swelling under and around the area are signs of something more serious than a strain. See an orthopedist.

What to do to recover:

- Treatment for strain
- RICE
- Use a compression (elastic) brace with a hole cut out to position the kneecap
- When range of motion and function return, rehab with weights

Osgoods Schlatta

This condition used to be called altar boys' knees from the large knobs of calcium that build up from kneeling for long periods. In this condition (often mis named a disease), the frontal thigh muscle (quadriceps) of a growing teenager is exerting too heavy a pull on its attachment point–the tibial tuberosity. This little mound of bone sits on the soft upper growth plate of the tibia and, as such, does not have a super strong attachment itself. When the muscle pulls and begins to tear the tibial tuberosity off of the plate, the body responds by bringing more calcium to the site in an attempt to "cement down" the tubercle. It is this that causes the "knob" to develop. As far as I know, no one has ever fully torn the tuberosity off the plate, though it is possible in theory. The pain in this condition comes from this tearing and from the strain at the patella tendon.

What to do to recover:

- RICE at least once a day, preferably right after practice or play
- Treatment for strain
- Use an Osgoods Schlatta knee strap during practice and play, or have the team athletic trainer tape the tibial tuberosity down

Dislocated Patella

Here we get into something called Q angle. The top of the rectus femoris muscle of the quadriceps group starts at the prominent bones at the front of the hips anterior superior pine of the

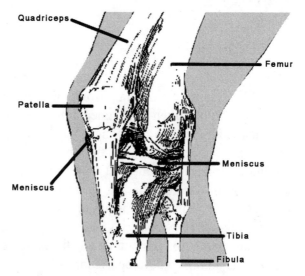

anterior pubic crest, if you need specifics. If you draw a straight line from there to the middle of the kneecap, you will have the line of pull of the quadriceps. Now from the middle of the kneecap continue that line to the tibial tuberosity where the patella ligament attaches south to the end of the quadriceps group and down. The straighter the line, the less will be the tendency to dislocate the kneecap. When angles of deviation approach 20 degrees or more, we call that an excessive Q angle.

Those athletes are likely to suffer occasional dislocations or subluxations (partial dislocations or dislocations that reduce themselves.)

Too much Q angle is seen mostly in women due to the structure of the hips and the medial (inward) inclination of the thigh bone as it goes to the leg. This creates an angle where the quadriceps wants to pull in as straight a line as it can. To do this, it has to reduce the Q angle, and it does this by drawing the kneecap out of its grove and over the knobs at the outer end of the knee joint. Ouch!

Many women start out with a "Patella Alta," or high placed kneecap. In other words, the patella ligament stretched during growth and the kneecap rides too far up on its groove (patella fossa). The fossa gets shallower as it goes up, and this predisposition makes it easier for the kneecap to slip out and travel to the outside.

Dislocations of the kneecap are easy to recognize, as the patella will obviously be out of place. Reducing the dislocation can be as easy as using thumb pressure from the outside to gently push the cap back to the center. If a dislocation has sat for too long unreduced, swelling will get in the way of reduction, and a physician must be seen to effect the reduction.

What to do to recover:

- Treatment for sprain
- RICE
- Obtain a patella tracking brace from a brace maker and always wear it during training and play

Fat Pad Injuries

Underneath the patella ligament and in front of the joint capsule lies an extra bit of protection in the form of a pad of fat. This poor forgotten structure gets kicked in soccer, pinched in hypertension injuries, mashed in falls onto the knee; everyone remembers the patella ligament and the bursa sacs above it, but no one remembers this fat pad until an injured athlete goes to take a step and straighten out the knee to, a nearly locking position catching the inside aspect of the pad between the upper and lower portions of the knee joint, that is! The pain is sharp, distinct, like a pinpoint and takes all of the steam out of the knee for a few seconds. Inflammation at the pad and the structures around it are the culprits causing the thing to go where it should not and get caught. This inflammation must be reduced.

What to do to recover:

- RICE
- Treatment for contusion
- Use a knee compression brace that also prevents full extension of the knee while the area is swollen

Rehab for Knee and Thigh Injuries

At times we want exercise with movement in the knee during rehab, and at times, like right after surgery, we don't. We will present simple versions of both types of these exercises here. Though it must be said that full range of motion usually cannot be achieved after surgery without the active help of an athletic trainer, exercise physiologist, or physical therapist. They have to physically force the knee to bend in order to break through he scar tissue that develops immediately after the operation.

Quad Setting

Sit on an exercise bench or treatment table with your back braced against the wall. The affected limb should be straight

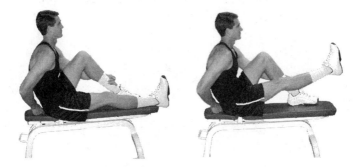

ahead of you and the other bent at the knee with the foot firmly placed on the table or bench. Keeping a straight knee, raise the affected limb until the foot is 8 to 12 inches off the bench. Hold and count to 20. Repeat 10 times do 3 sets.

Partial Knee Extensions

For those with kneecap injuries the most painful part of the range of motion is the middle of straightening the knee. In early

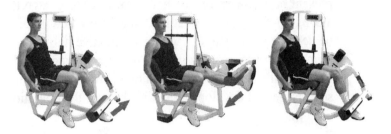

knee rehab often partial movement is done for exercise. Here we will do the upper 1/3 of the knee extension movement for 3

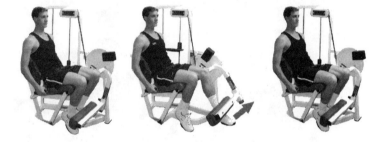

sets of 5 to 7 reps and then the lower 1/3 of the movement for the same amount of work. Not all weightlifting or resistance gear is capable of such movement so machines that will accommodate the movement must be found.

Full Knee Extensions

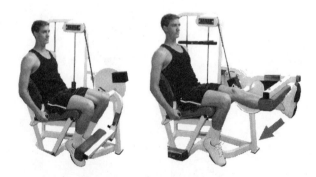

Knee Flexion

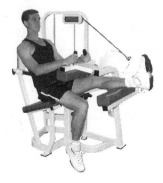
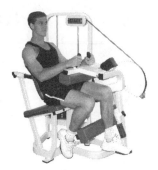

Quad Stretch

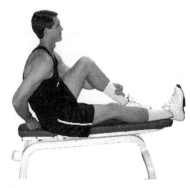
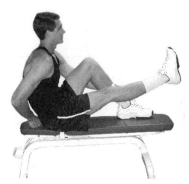

Seated Toe Reach

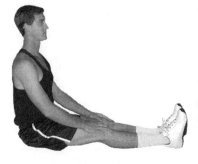
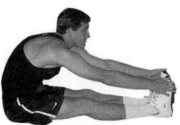

NOTES

NOTES

NOTES

Chapter 9
Hip, Pelvis, and Lower Back Injuries

• • • • • •

We deal with these areas as a group due to their mechanical interrelation. For example, several muscles of the groin and frontal hip are actually also lower back muscles! The outward rotators of the hip muscles attach to the borders of the sacrum and thus effect the lower back and its nerves.

First let's cover the bony anatomy of the area. The pelvis is a basin, and, as such, it holds the reproductive organs, urinary bladder, and much of the intestines. Aside from what's inside, it also serves as the connecting point for the

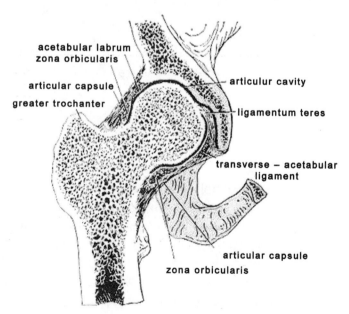

acetabular labrum
zona orbicularis

articular capsule
greater trochanter

articulur cavity

ligamentum teres

transverse – acetabular ligament

articular capsule
zona orbicularis

Coronal section of right hip–showing articular cavity and capsule

thigh bones. These attach at the hip joint. This deep and strong joint is held in place by the Y-shaped ilio-femoral ligament, the strongest and thickest ligament of the body.

At the rear of the pelvic basin sits the sacrum. This triangular bone, nestled apex, down in the back of the iliac crest is held in place by the ilio-sacral ligaments. The sacrum is a semi-moveable joint, and aside from having the rest of the spine sit on it, it also forms the bottom of the cerebral spinal fluid pump. Brain and spinal fluid circulate to provide the outer portions of the central nervous system with oxygen. Two bones that form the floor of the scull, the sphenoid and the occiput, form the top of the pump. When we breathe, the scull bones raise almost

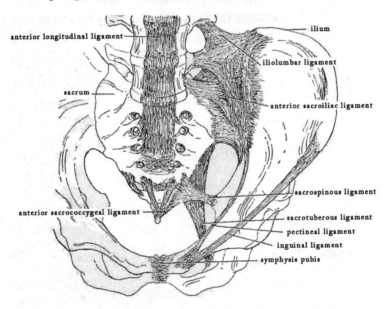

imperceptibly at their central joint under the brain. This pumps the fluid around the brain and down the spinal canal. In the same breath, the sacrum teeter-totters a minute amount front to back and pumps the fluid back. If either one of the pumps is not working due to injury, inflammation, or restriction, headaches at the base of the scull will result. These headaches can be tremendously bad and crippling.

Below the sacrum is a tiny bone called the coccyx, known commonly as the tailbone. This little guy is so covered and wrapped around by nerves that any little boo-boo feels like a major injury, and is unbearably painful. Ask anyone who has ever had one dislocated by a kick or any mother who fractured one during childbirth!

Sitting atop the sacrum are the lumbar vertebrae of the spinal column. These hard-working spinal bones bear the weight of all you do. Between these bones are jelly doughnut-like structures known as the inter vertebral disks. They deepen the joints allowing greater movement between the articulations and acting as shock absorbers. When they are squeezed too hard, the jelly (nucleus pulposa) in the middle ruptures, oozing out putting pressure on the nerves beneath it, causing the pain of a ruptured disk. To understand how this mechanism works, next time you have a jelly doughnut to spare, put it between your two fists and squeeze the fists together at one end. The jelly will come shooting out the other side. That's exactly how disks bulge and herniate.

Most Common Injuries

Contusions to the Genitalia

Hits here are very painful for women as well as for men. Both sexes have an abundant nerve supply to the external genitalia, and these nerves of pleasure can transmit pain signals as well. The sensory nerve supply here is so rich and so sensitive that little hurts feel like big hurts, and big hurts feel unbearable.

In both sexes contusions to these organs can cause swelling. In men this swelling can become extreme and create a condition known as hydroseal. In this malady swelling, coupled with inflamed tissue, creates a compartment syndrome similar to that of the leg, trapping an increasing amount of fluid which becomes very painful and very dangerous. If the swelling is not reduced by aspiration, death of tissue (necrosis) can result. If it is ignored long enough, gangrene can set in. If you're not suffering with this condition, the thought of piercing the scrotum (testicle sac) with a big needle is repulsive to most men. In the case of hydroseal, however, the needle is a welcome sight, and pales when compared to the pain of the swelling.

If the blow is strong enough, a testicle may rupture (explode). Pain from a strike to the groin that lasts more than a few minuets and is accompanied by swelling of the scrotum, may cause serious damage – get that man to the emergency room quickly.

Most testicle pain that occurs after a hit can be attributed to a spasm in the levator testi muscles. This is the little set of muscles that raise and lower the testicles. When these guys go into a spasm, the pain is tremendous. Aside from actually reaching down and pulling the testicles away from the pelvis, the most common way to relieve testicular spasm in sports is the following:

Have the athlete sit straight-legged on the ground with the feet slightly apart and arms crossed along the chest. From behind, the trainer, coach, or interested individual lifts the athlete's fanny up some 8 inches by pulling up from the armpits and then summarily dropping him. This is repeated several times until the spasm eases. Here we have a simple physics lesson. When the pelvis hits the ground, the testicles continue on their downward travel to stretch the levator testi, and this stretches the muscles.

What to do to recover:

- Seek medical attention if pain and swelling persist
- RICE
- Treatment for contusion

Internal Pelvic Injuries

Most of the internal organs housed by the pelvis are safe from all but the hardest blunt trauma suffered by athletics. While mild contusions are common, more serious injuries are infrequent. The serious ones are usually caused by a kick, a helmet spear, or a fall onto equipment. The most common of these is the ruptured urinary bladder.

Ruptured Urinary Bladder. Going out onto the field or court with a full or semi-full bladder is inviting trouble. Imagine carrying a water-filled balloon around in front of you while you run, jump, kick, or play. What happens if that balloon takes a hit? You bet, it blows up. That's just about what happens when the bladder ruptures. As you can imagine, it is not pleasant and will take a bit of surgery to correct.

The signs of serious abdominal or internal pelvic injury are: pain, abdominal rigidity, and possibly fever. Don't monkey with the "what ifs." If the hit was hard and there is pain, get to an emergency room.

What to do to recover:

- Medical treatment
- RICE
- Treatment for contusion
- Rehab and strengthen the area with weights

External Pelvic Injuries

Hip Pointers. These are bruises to the top of the iliac crest where the oblique muscles connect to the bone. While not dangerous or life-threatening, they cause pain and impair movement. If the contusion produces extended pain or a mild grinding sensation, x-rays must be taken to determine if the crest has been fractured.

What to do to recover:

- RICE.
- Wear back belt
- Treatment for contusion

Hip Dislocations. Thankfully, these are rare in sports. The Y ligament is so strong that in most instances, it prevents the ball from coming out of the socket. In some folks the socket is shallower than in others and the Y ligament is not as strong. The athlete will have an obvious deformity at the hip when it is dislocated. Call for an ambulance and transport the athlete to the hospital. Usually these dislocations are difficult to reset and reduction, under anesthesia, may be necessary.

What to do to recover:

- RICE
- Treatment for Sprain

Acetabular Fractures. Forces pushing the ball part of the thigh bone hard into the joint sometimes cracks the hip socket. Any deep lingering pain needs to be evaluated by an orthopedist. Warning signs that there may be a problem include the inability to bear weight, grinding sensations or sounds, or deep and persistent pain.

What to do to recover:

- Seek orthopedic evaluation
- RICE
- Treatment for contusion

Aseptic Necrosis of the Hip Joint. Even fully conditioned players cannot get around their genetic limitations. Some folks have very little in the way of blood vessels to the hip joint. And while it is true that exercise can increase the size and number of blood vessels in any muscular area, the deep hip joint is comprised of bones, tendons, ligaments, and synovial (lubrication) membranes. None of these tissues benefits from the increase in vascularization of conditioned muscles. In other words, there is no increase in circulation to the hip joint in people who have a lack of blood supply there.

There have been a couple of famous cases where star pro athletes were suddenly knocked out of their playing lives by the death of the tissue deep in the hip joint. Hip replacements are necessary in these cases because the bone and cartilage of the ball and socket die. Running backs and home run hitters have a hard time running on stainless steel and plastic; it just can't measure up to the original thing! This is a carrier-ending condition.

What to do to recover:

- After surgery, RICE
- Treatment for fracture
- Treatment for sprain
- Use post op treatment plan
- Rehabilitate professionally to regain full use

Sacroiliac Joint Subluxation. This is likely the most common pelvic condition. Here the Sacroiliac (SI) joints formed by the iliac crest connecting to and nestling the sacrum become slightly dislocated (subluxated). The condition is very painful, can be very crippling, and is the easiest thing in the world (for someone who knows how) to correct. Once that's done, the pain and dysfunction is instantly gone! Pain at the pelvis on one of the "dimples" just outside the lumbar spine and sacrum indicate sacroiliac joint problem. The experts here are the chiropractors. Do not go to an MD for this condition, or you may find yourself having unnecessary surgery. Many orthopedists can't tell the difference between a lower lumbar injury and a sacroiliac subluxation. It sounds utterly stupid that they don't, but most don't, that herniated disks are the two most missed diagnoses MDs make with regard to the back.

Since there is little muscle at this site, all the lower back and abdomen strengthening won't help or prevent the SI joint from popping out if the forces against it are just right.

What to do to recover:

- Get chiropractic treatment
- RICE
- Treatment for sprain

Lumbar Spine Injuries

Boo-boos here run the gamut from mild sprains of the interconnecting ligament of the lower spine to straining the muscle surrounding them to subluxations and ruptured disks. There are so many parts and pieces down there that experts need to be consulted to properly diagnose the damage. Here again the Doctor of Chiropractic (DC) is superior to the orthopedist in training and technique. Who would you rather see for treatment of this area, someone who studied the spine for 4 solid years or someone who studied the area for only a few weeks or months? (Yes, I said weeks. Look over medical school curriculums and you'll see this old professor of physical medicine is right!)

Some things all back injuries have in common. In all cases of back pain spasm, only 4 muscle groups cause most of the pain. These muscles are the Ilio-Posas group, the Quadratus Lumborum, the Pyriformis, and the Ilio-tibial band (ITB). If these muscles are released from their deep spasm, most pain, even sciatic pain, will be greatly relieved. Luckily, we only need two stretches to release these afflicted muscles.

- Hip Roll Stretch
- Single Knee to Chest stretch

The Hip Roll Stretch. This is the only effective stretch for the pesky pyriformis muscle that bears down on the sciatic nerve and causes it to hurt. It also effectively stretches the quadratus and ITB. Follow the picture. Keep the shoulders flat during the stretch and allow the knee and foot to drop toward the floor. Do 3 stretches to one side holding each stretch for 40 seconds; then change position and do 3 to the other side. Take each stretch only to the first point of pain, no further. As you progress, that first point of pain will occur further and further into the stretch.

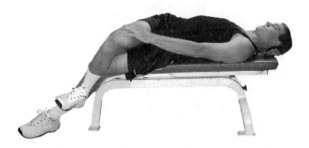

Single Knee to Chest Stretch. Here draw one knee up to the chest while allowing the other to dangle freely from the hip off the corner or edge of a bed or bench. Again bring the knee up only to the first point of pain and hold for 40 seconds. Repeat 3 times on either side.

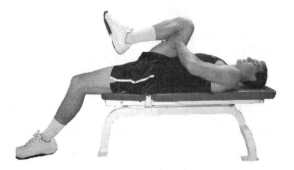

Get all lumbar injuries checked out by a good DC, then rehab and treat as below.

What to do to recover:

- Chiropractic care
- RICE
- Hip roll stretch 3 x 40 seconds per stretch
- Single knee stretch 3 x 40 seconds per stretch
- Treatment for sprain
- When ready for rehabilitation, do 45 degree roman chair back extensions

Rehab for Lower Back Injuries

By far the most common of work related injuries. Back trauma may come on suddenly as the result of a particular event, usually, a bad lift. Back injuries may also be the cumulative effect of little hurts. Regardless, these injuries range in intensity from mild strains to near crippling herniation of the intervertebral disks. Many of the stretching and strengthening programs used in physical therapy were developed by people who were not completely familiar with human bio-mechanics. (Kinesiology is not taught in P.T. school. Neither is work / exercise physiology, though both are intimately related to the work that must be done with orthopedic patients). It also is apparent that those who develop these programs never had any back pain.

There may be several sources of back pain. First, there is the pain of the injured tissue. In a sprain or strain, soft tissue tears produce pain. In sacroiliac joint subluxation, the ligaments and other soft tissue around the joint get stretched and pinched, producing tremendous pain added to the structural instability caused by the malposition itself. Another type of pain especially in the front of the groin, the front of the thigh, and the leg as spinal nerve trunks are pressed by the jelly from burst intervertebral disks.

In any back condition the injury is made worse by the negative reaction of four large muscle groups. These muscles spasm in an attempt to splint the area, preventing further movement which the body thinks would bring further damage. It's these muscle groups that either cause pain within themselves from the spasm or press down on nearby nerves, causing rivers of radiating pain. This is what happens in sciatica, which is secondary pain associated with many back conditions.

The Ilio-posas, the Quadratus Lumborum, the Piriformis, and the Ilio-Tibial band are the spasming quartet that worsen the pain of back injuries. These muscles, and the paraspinals above them, also try to put the body into a less painful walking and standing position (antalgia) resulting in the twisted postures seen in patients with acute back problems. The problem with antalgic conditions is that we get used to the twists, and if the pain is present long enough, i.e. weeks or months, those kinks may become more or less a permanent part of our posture and gait. This will then create problems of its own. So what's to be done?

Stretching

Be forewarned that stretching is not easy or pain free. A good stretch directly involving spasm or contractured (abnormally shortened) muscles will hurt like the dickens. The trick in stretching is to take a stretching position to its first point of pain, hold it there, then count slowly to 30, relaxing along the way. A muscle taken past its accustomed range of motion will react by involuntarily contracting (stretch reflex). This initial contraction usually releases in about 20 seconds; it's only after that release that you're really stretching. When you hit 30, return to the pre-stretch position, rest 10 seconds, and repeat the stretch. Do each stretch 4 times. This stretching program should be done first thing in the morning before arising from bed, the last thing at night, and any time in the middle of the day if you feel stiff or experience the onset of pain from spasm.

Essential Stretch #1: Hip Roll

This stretch is for the Quadratus Lumborum, Piriformis, and Ilio-Tibial Band. Lie flat on your bed. Now turn the hips to point the one furthest from the edge at the ceiling. Then bend that hip and knee 90 degrees and rotate the foot down toward the floor. Ouch! Yes, that's it; you've got it! That pain across the buttocks is the little muscle called the piriformis. That's the guy that presses down on the sciatic nerve and causes that intense pain. Allowing the leg to rotate down toward the floor intensifies the stretch on the piriformis, taking it out of spasm. This movement hurts, but it does wonders to relieve sciatic pain! Hold for 30 seconds; roll back until flat on the bed. Rest, and

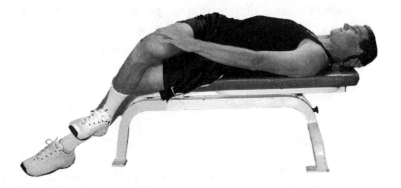

repeat in 10 seconds. Then slide over to the other edge of the bed and stretch the other side. You will notice that one side will hurt and be less flexible than the other; this is normal and caused by the lateral (side) injury.

Essential Stretch #2: Single Knee to Chest Stretch

This stretches the Ilio-Posas, the Gluteals, the Hamstrings, and the lumbar Paraspinals. Bring your hips to the edge of your bed. With both legs hanging down to the floor, take one knee in both hands and draw it up toward your chest as far as you can bring it. Let the other leg hang. At the first point of pain hold that position and count to 30. When that stretch is done, let that knee down and do the other side. Do each side 4 times. Make sure that you allow the bottom leg to hang.

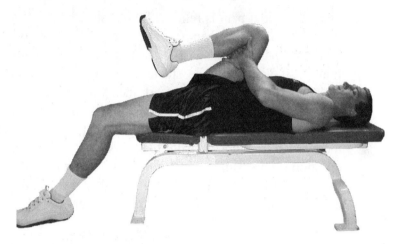

This is the most important part of this stretch as when the limb is hanging you are pulling the Ilio-Posas directly. It is that muscle that shortens giving the duck-like lordotic position to our stance. That position, aside from being painful, squeezes the posterior aspects of the lumbar disks forcing more of their soft insides to go forward against the nerve trunks, or worse, against the neural canal (which houses the spinal chord). When shortened, the Ilio-Posas is notorious for straining and tearing, causing a good bit of pain. As you progress in this stretch, the knee will come further back toward your chest, and the lower leg will get closer to the floor and have less tendency to hike up at the hip as you pull on the opposite knee.

After these two stretches, take 2 minutes to massage each foot, especially around the arch. This action opens the circulation to your back and lower extremities. The arch lies over the vessels of venous and lymphatic return. When the tissues there are stiff and short from sleeping, our ability to circulate blood to the back and legs will be impeded for as long as it takes us to warm up. Try this experiment. One morning after your stretches, massage one foot and not the other; then stand up. See how your legs feel. I guarantee that you will sit back down and massage the other foot!

Once the initial pain is relieved by our stretching routine, you need to start strengthening your back. It's not too early. Atrophy (muscle wastage and shrinkage) sets in rapidly after injury. If you are to be stable and get through your daily activities without too much effort, then you need to work at it. Not maintaining a good strengthening program will relegate you to future back injuries sooner! All back patients will re-injure their backs. That is a given due to the instability of the area. The question is how badly and for how long? A strong and flexible back will sustain lower levels of injury than a weak, tight one, and the stronger back will bounce back sooner than a frail one.

Low Back Strengthening Progression

Working on the lower back muscles at first requires no fancy equipment. Nothing other than an empty piece of floor and a pillow. These exercises need only be done 3 to 4 times a week. Since strength exercise involves a different physiological response than stretching, overdoing strength exercises by performing them too often can work against what you are trying to accomplish.

Prone Hyperextension Level A

Lie face down on the floor with a pillow under your front hip bones as shown. Your chin is centered on the deck, your hands

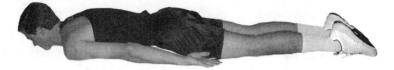

at your side. Slowly raise your chin, shoulders, and chest from the floor. Once your chest is some 4 inches up, stop and go back to the starting position. Be sure to exhale on the way up and

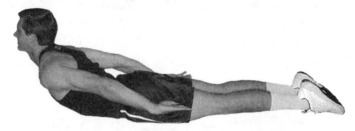

inhale on the way down. Try to do 8. Rest for a minute, then do 8 more. In total, do 3 sets of 8 repetitions. Every week you will add 2 repetitions to each set until you hit 16 reps – then proceed to Level B of this exercise.

Prone Hyperextension Level B

Lie face down as above. This time when you lift your shoulders simultaneously lift the knees and feet from the floor some 4 to 6 inches. Breathe out on lifting, in on the way back to the floor.

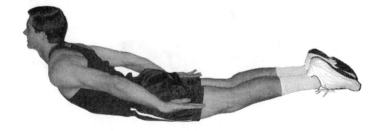

You don't have to hold the topmost position. Move slowly, but as soon as you get there move back down again. Progress on the repetitions as you did above.

Prone Hyperextensions, Levels C and D.

After the week of 3 sets of 16 reps level B, move your hands

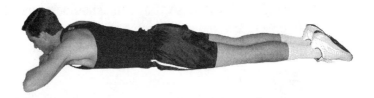

under your chest (level C) as shown and begin the progression

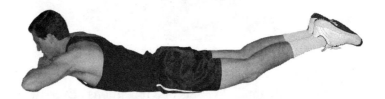

again. In level D (below), the arms are straight out as shown. The progression remains the same.

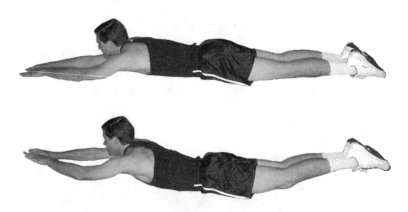

Abdominal strength forms the body's natural supportive girdle. It's not enough to have a set of strong lower back muscles if the other muscles of the midsection don't support the back in its actions.

Crunch Sit-ups Level A

Lie face up, back flat on the floor with your hips and knees bent. Place your hands palms down on your thighs. Slide your

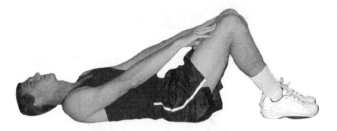

fingertips toward the kneecaps, lift your head and shoulders 4 to 6 inches off of the ground, and breathe out. Slide back and

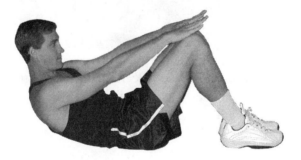

repeat. Do 3 sets of 8 to 16 repetitions with a minute or two of rest between each set.

Note: At first some folks feel this exercise more in the front of the neck than in the abdomen; this means your neck muscles are in a sorrier state than your tummy. To minimize this stress, tuck your chin lightly toward your chest and hold this position through the set.

Crunch Sit-ups Level B

Lie on your back face up with the same knee and hip position as you did previously. This time, instead of holding your hands on

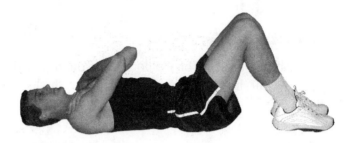

your lap, cross your arms over your chest. Perform the exercise as you did before but as you've changed the leverage, it will be

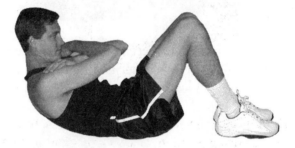

more difficult to do. Decrease the repetitions and progress through them as you did before from 3 sets of 8 to 3 sets of 16 by adding 2 reps per week to each set.

Crunch Sit Ups Level C

Now you're playing with the grown-ups. Place your hands under your neck and throughout the movement keep your elbows out to the sides so as not to pull on your head and crane your neck forward. Progress through your sets from fewer repetitions to more only this time don't stop adding reps at 16. Add two reps a week for a year! This will leave you somewhere at 3 sets of some 200 reps per set. This will give you an abdomen that can shield you against injury – if you remember to use it. Many folks have good abdominal strength but forget to tighten their tummies when lifting and, in so doing, leave the

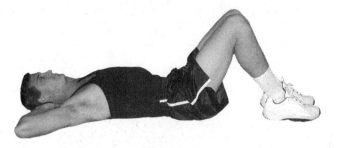

back to work alone, unshielded and unsupported. This will result in injury.

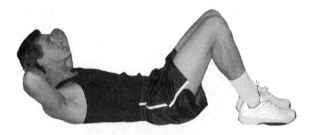

Note: If your lower back is uncomfortable or even painful in the regular sit-up position, place a light chair by your feet, put your heels on the chair, and snug yourself in toward the chair. The bio-mechanical rule here is that the closer your knees are to your shoulders with your lumbars flat, the safer and more pain free your back will be through the sit up movement.

● ● ● ● ● ●

NOTES

Chapter 10
Abdominal and Torso Injuries
• • • • • •

Most of us think that merely by having a perfect set of abdominal muscles keeps us from ever falling victim to abdominal injuries. While it's true that having six-pack abs goes a long way to protect the midsection and what's inside, they don't always afford the protection one would think.

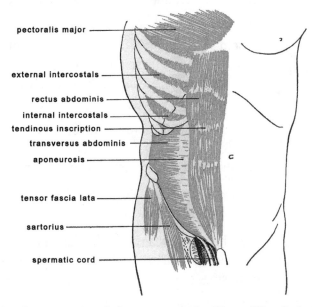

pectoralis major

external intercostals

rectus abdominis

internal intercostals

tendinous inscription

transversus abdominis

aponeurosis

tensor fascia lata

sartorius

spermatic cord

Take the example of the escape artist Harry Houdini. He had such a magnificent set of abdominal muscles that he would challenge circus strongmen and professional boxers to hit him there. Once he would contract his abs, he could take a hit there just fine. But once, just once, a strongman punched him in the stomach before he was ready – that cost

Houdini his life. Abs cannot always be tight and contracted. (Even the most conceited bodybuilder can't keep his abs sucked in and tight 24/7). During play the discipline of tightening the gut can be forgotten in the mad rush of activity and despite our best conditioning, injuries occur.

Most Common Injuries

Contusion of the Abdomen or Celiac (Solar) Plexus

Most folks are familiar with getting the wind knocked out of them. A heavy blow to the abdomen causes a reflex in the diaphragm and momentarily prevents breathing. This is followed by the familiar gasping for air as the diaphragm spasm subsides. During the "I can't breathe phase," calm the player, loosen his belt, and reassure him that relaxing will restore his breath faster. Have the injured athlete breathe in short little breaths at first until the spasm is totally gone.

Once the breathless phase is over, the bottom of the sternum should be examined by health personnel to determine if the xyphiod has been fractured. The xyphiod is a small and fragile bone that, if broken and pushed back, can lacerate the liver and cause internal bleeding.

If the athlete fails to begin breathing or his lips turn blue (cyanosis), mouth to mouth resuscitation should be administered until emergency medical help arrives.

Abdominal rigidity and pain are likely signs of internal injuries, get emergency medical help fast.

The abdominals can be bruised as can any muscle that has been strained or contused; the soft tissue should be treated for contusion.

What to do to recover:

- If breathing does not improve, get medical help and start mouth to mouth resuscitation
- Relax and reassure the patient
- Check for xyphoid fracture
- Treatment for contusion

Rupture of the Spleen

Aside from kidney failure, ruptured spleens are a leading cause of death from athletics. The spleen is a gelatinous-like organ which has various functions. It can act as a reservoir for blood. At sleep and during rest when the physiological demands of the body are low, the spleen and liver hold up to 1/3 of the body's blood supply. The stitch in the side often felt by beginning runners is sometimes the result of the spleen squeezing itself to put more blood into circulation to meet the new demand for oxygen. The spleen is also involved with immunity, producing white blood cells and destroying old ineffective blood cells.

The spleen is soft and gelatinous-like, making it a good candidate for rupture from a heavy blow. The external sign of a ruptured spleen is called Kerrs Sign and evidences itself as pain along the inside of the left ribcage and chest, up the armpit and the inside of the arm. Many folks mistake it for the pain from a heart attack. But the pain along the inside of the armpit and arm are the giveaways.

After a blow, the spleen can do a good job of bandaging itself with a patch of more gelatin-like substance, but the slightest thing can force the patch from its tenuous position and, boom, you have a gusher of blood filling the abdominal cavity. These patches have been known to come off days or weeks after the event that caused the rupture. Depending on the size of the rupture, it's possible to bleed within death in hours, or even minutes. Kerrs Sign should not be ignored or "walked off." These are not any symptoms to play with. Get medical help immediately.

What to do to recover:

- Get medical attention immediately
- After surgery - Post Operative Recovery Treatment for 6 months
- Do not resume play, training, or practice until medically cleared to do so

Cardiac Contusion

This is a bruise to the heart muscle. As simple and harmless as that sounds, it is far from it. In bruises, tissues swell; swelling causes pressure changes within the tissue and a lessening of function. The greater the bruise, the lower the function – are you getting my drift? Unlike your bicep that can stop all action and take it easy when it gets hurt, <u>your heart can't do that</u>. **If it stops to rest, you're dead.**

If a heavy blow to the sternum, or just below, brings on chest pain accompanied by shortness of breath, the need to cough in order to breathe, light headedness, dizziness, blue lips, or the traditional heart attack scenario of chest pain radiating to the shoulder and the arm, get to an ER, pronto!

Once you're home, treat your heart muscle for inflammation. Since you can't put an ice bag on your heart, use plenty of systemic enzymes.

What to do to recover:

- Rest, Rest, Rest
- Enzymes, Enzymes, Enzymes
- Treatment for contusion
- Continue rest and treatment until medically cleared to return to play

Kidney Contusions

The kidneys are located on either side of your thoracic spine. The top half are cradled by the lower ribs while the bottom half have no bony protection. Because these organs filter gunk out of your blood, they are always engorged with blood. It's doesn't take a rocket scientist or a kidney surgeon to see that if you bump a swollen water balloon hard enough, it's going to burst! And while burst is not exactly what these puppies do, they <u>do</u> rupture their membranes and bleed. The degree of injury depends on the force of the blow and the angle at which it is received.

Aside from the mid-back pain, those with kidney contusions may display signs of shock, nausea or vomiting, spasm or rigidity in the back muscles, and blood in the urine. Someone displaying any or all of these symptoms needs to see a doctor immediately. Bedrest for observation is usually recommended to see if the bleeding stops on its own. If the damage is extensive, though, surgery may be needed.

What to do to recover:

- Get medical attention
- Treatment for contusion after the observation period, if bleeding stops by itself
- Get medical clearance before resuming work, training, or play

Rib Fractures

While most rib fractures occur from a blow to the chest during a contact sport, they can also occur via "indirect trauma" such as a violent muscular contraction, or even from coughing. Direct trauma displaces the ribs inwardly toward the internal organs. This is the most dangerous type fracture as the jagged broken ends can tear and perforate the chest lining (pleurae), lungs, liver, kidneys, etc. seriously compounding the injury.

Rib fractures are quite easy to detect, but unless you know what to palpate or test for, it's best to leave things alone; transport the person to the emergency room, and let the doctors earn their keep. Fractures here usually heal in 3 to 4 weeks.

What to do to recover:

- Get medical evaluation
- Treatment for fracture
- Do not play until medical clearance has been given
- Rehabilitate Chest and Upper / Mid Back areas with weights

Subluxated Rib Heads

This common condition often causes piercing, burning pain just to the side of the spine where the ribs connect. MDs, unfamiliar with the condition often mistake this pain for a muscle tear or some sort of spinal injury. The pain comes from the slight dislocation of the head of the rib from the small notch it's supposed to ride in. Once the rib head is out of place, it presses on all of the soft tissue that surrounds it sending the rich sensory nerves suppling those tissues with sensory perception into a frenzy of pain. If the spasm resulting from the subluxations is not too bad, the rib heads may be put back in using the following technique.

Hang from a chinning bar, count slowly to 30, breathe deeply, and relax. Between the stretch's pull and release, you might feel the mild clunk of the bones popping back into place. Most of the time, though, the resulting spasm in the surrounding muscular tissue will be so bad that it will need a chiropractor, osteopath or naturopath to adjust the bones and put the ribs back in. Pain relief is instantaneous once the subluxation has been reduced.

What to do to recover:

- See a Chiropractor, Naturopath or Osteopath to have the bones reseated
- Treatment for sprain

Costochondral Cartilage Separation

Though few have heard of this injury, it actually occurs more often than rib fractures. The ribs do not have a bony connection

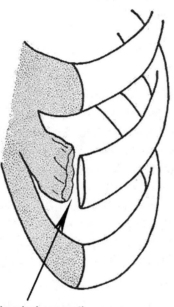

costochondral separation

to the sternum (breastbone). Since the area has a lot of give and take, the articulation between these bones must be a flexible one. Finger-like projections emanate from the sides of the breastbone for a few inches and then attach to the ends of the ribs. The same mechanisms that bring about fractured ribs, when applied to the front of the chest, can cause the cartilage to tear off of the rib end. There will be pinpoint pain at the front of the chest and often, if the tear is complete, the rib will stick out like an unbound spring.

While most orthopedists these days choose not to repair the unsightly rib which protrudes, the repair is easily affected as same day surgery and involves a small incision, drilling two holes, and tying the lose ends together with stainless steel wire. Most doctors today try bracing the rib cage with an elastic bandage and hope that the ends come close enough together to mend. Wishful thinking! You've got to take the brace off sometimes, even if only to shower. When the tension is gone, the rib will pop out again. If minor surgery is not performed, the injury will heal much more slowly, resulting in a rib that continues to protrude. In a man it looks odd, for a woman it can be devastating. Find an orthopedic surgeon who knows how to fix it, and get the job done right!

What to do to recover:

- Get medical attention
- Treatment for fracture
- Treatment for strain
- Get the area repaired

Injuries to the Lungs

The power of falls, tackles, and strikes is absorbed by the chest and can cause a variety of extremely serious injuries to the lungs. Broken ribs that rip into the chest cavity will damage the inner chest wall (pleurae), allowing air to get into the cavity. The lung cavity normally has negative pressure; in other words, it has a vacuum inside. This allows the lungs to fill with air. If there was air already in the cavity, the lungs could not expand. When the inner chest wall tears, air gets sucked into the lung and that side collapses. It then looks like an airless deflated balloon. This is called Pneumothorax. (Pneumos is Greek for breath or spirit.) In first aid this is called a sucking chest wound.

If a blow has caused bleeding within the pleural cavity and fills with blood, the lung cannot expand. This is known as a Hemothorax. (Hemo means blood.) Both the Pneumothorax and the Hemothorax are caused by rib fractures pushing in and tearing things up.

A very dangerous condition that can occur to the lungs without a rib fracture is a Lung Hemorrhage. Here a violent blow compresses the lungs and ruptures its tissue. Internal bleeding occurs in the lungs causing difficulty breathing and the pain associated with it. Frothy blood is coughed up.

Needless to say, someone needs to dial 911 immediately when it comes to these injuries.

What to do to recover:

- Get medical help
- After surgery use the Post Operative Recovery Treatment
- Treatment for strain
- If blood loss has been great, treatment for contusion and hemorrhage

Miscellaneous Strains

There are a lot of muscles from the bellybutton to the clavicle – and all are subject to straining. Don't ignore anything that lasts longer than a day. More than momentary loss of function, strength, or ROM, denotes a more serious injury than a 1st degree. Any popping heard during the injury or any creaking or clicking in an area after an injury are all red flashing lights. Get them checked out.

What to do to recover:

- Get medical evaluation
- Treatment for strain

NOTES

NOTES

NOTES

Chapter 11
Shoulder Injuries
● ● ● ● ● ●

The first thing to remember about shoulder injuries is that little injuries hurt like big injuries and big injuries are unbelievably painful. This is due to the rich blood supply coming to the a group of nerves known as the Brachial Plexus, which lie in the armpit (axial). If only the muscles in the shoulder were as well fed as these nerves, recovery from surgery wouldn't take such a long time.

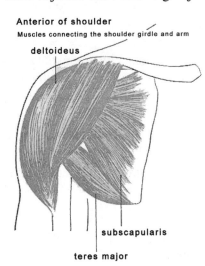

Anterior of shoulder
Muscles connecting the shoulder girdle and arm
deltoideus
subscapularis
teres major

At the shoulder we have two joints, one semi-movable and one fully movable. The shoulder girdle, comprised of the sternum, the clavicle, and the scapula, forms the "yardarm" that allows our upper extremities to have the range of motion around

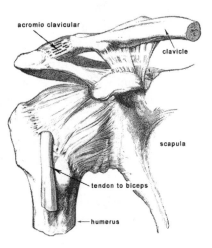

acromio clavicular
clavicle
scapula
tendon to biceps
humerus

our torsos. The shoulder joint is what most folks think of as the shoulder. This area consists of the ball or the upper arm bone (Humerus) and the socket of the scapula (wing bone).

Injuries to the Shoulder Girdle

Acromio Clavicular Joint Separations

First, let's take a look at the arrangement of the shoulder girdle and its weak points. The only thing holding this yardarm arrangement to the rest of the skeleton is the ligament located on the inner portion of the clavicle where the upper part of the sternum meets the manubrium bone. The outer end of the clavicle and the wing bone have no connection to the rest of the skeleton at all. This allows the yardarm to move freely up, down, in, out, and across. The weak point here is the articulation of the clavicle with the scapula (Acromio Clavicular or AC joint.) Though the ligament holding the AC joint is very strong, it can, over time, be overworked. Worse yet, a blow can cause it to separate. This separation may be partial or full but is painful in either case. The usual test for a separated shoulder is to tap two finger tips right on the point formed by the acromio clavicular joint. If the joint is injured, the pain brought on by tapping is enough to bring a fully grown football player to his knees.

In partial separations, the arms and shoulder are placed in a cross brace which pulls the bones closer together to allow them to mend in a position closer to the original. This brace is worn during the day for 6 weeks. If the truth be known however, I've seldom seen it work! In full separations the last outer inch of the clavicle is surgically sawed off, to what end I haven't yet figured out. That leaves nothing but muscle holding up the mast and that is just stupid. Muscle is supposed to make things move, not hold things together. Joints are supposed to move around a pivot, so what happens when you cut off the pivot and leave structures hanging freely?

The old way of fixing AC joint separations is much better in terms of time spent out of action (a few days as opposed to 6 to 8 weeks) and makes much better biomechanical sense than chopping of the head of the joint! The old repair is made with a small incision over the site. Then a small hole is drilled through both the clavicle and the acromion of the scapula through which stainless steel wire is threaded, and the joint drawn back together. This allows the area to heal with the bones touching, and a nearly instant return to activity. What is ultimately best is that this repair leaves the joint intact. There is some restriction in outward rotation because the wire does not allow the clavicle to fully turn on the acromion, but the restriction is minor and the downside negligible when compared to the alternative – removing the joint altogether!!!

Why is the joint-chopping procedure used? For only two reasons that I can figure:

The first reason is it costs more money. Remember orthopedists are, above all, surgeons, and surgeons cut things. The more they cut the better. The longer, more involved, and the more complicated the procedure, the more they and the rest of the medical staff can get involved and collect. Don't believe for a second that most doctors here will be satisfied with a good cheep fix – 80% of them won't.

Doing the most for the least is the order of the day in Europe where it costs society money when someone is sick or injured. Stateside, the medical system does not make any money unless someone gets sick or injured and they can prescribe grandiose treatments, sometimes even slowing your progress to keep charging the insurance company. I'm not making this up...I've had both MDs and chiropractors complain that the patients they sent to me were getting better too quickly, and, as a result, they were not getting to charge for enough visits and services!

The second reason why chopping is favored is because of a word I used earlier, Biomechanics. MDs never study it! Remarkable! One would think that orthopedic and reconstructive surgeons would be experts at biomechanics. Not a chance. They pick up some knowledge along the way, but as far as formal learning of biomechanics at school in class goes – it never happens, not in any medical school in the US. Most any undergraduate Physical

Education majors know a damn sight more about biomechanics than most orthopedic surgeons! It happens that the only doctors with training in biomechanics are those who have earned pervious degrees in Physical Education, Exercise Science, or Kinesiology (the formal name for biomechanics). So the chopping off procedure is the result of a lack of formal education with regard to the purpose, actions, and functions of joints in sports and life! Sad.

What to do to recover:

- Get medical attention
- RICE
- Treatment for sprain
- Do not train upper body, or play, until cleared by physician
- Train with weights to restore muscle mass lost to atrophy

Sterno Clavicular Separations

The next most frequently seen injury to the shoulder girdle involves separation of the clavicle from the sternum (Sterno Clavicular joint or SC). This is an extremely painful injury, very obvious to the eye, and easily corrected by manipulation. After the inner head of the clavicle is again situated in its notch on the clavicle, the patient is put in a brace which is very similar to the AC separation brace for a period of several weeks. There will be a tendency toward continued slippage and subluxation if the period of bracing does not promote full healing. Here again a little bit of stainless steel wire does wonders as does a less invasive treatment called prolotherapy. In prolotherapy, ligaments are injected with a saline solution meant to create a scarring reaction at the ligament. This scarring of the ligament increases its mass and strengthens and tightens it. It is the only non-surgical method available to repair partial ligament tears and loose ligaments. These days mostly osteopaths perform this wonderful therapy.

What to do to recover:

- Get medical attention
- RICE
- Treatment for sprain
- Do not train upper body, or play, until cleared by physician
- Train with weights to restore muscle mass lost to atrophy

Clavicular Fractures

A blow to the shaft of the clavicle can cause this bone to fracture. Football and the grappling sports (i.e., judo, jujitsu, acid, and wrestling) are the most likely places one will see this injury. Setting the bone straight is not a problem, but casting it is. Usually a partial body cast that covers the upper torso is the order of the day for about 12 to 16 weeks.

What to do to recover:

- Get medical attention
- RICE
- Treatment for sprain
- Do not train upper body, or play, until cleared by physician
- Train with weights to restore muscle mass lost to atrophy

Shoulder Girdle Muscle Injuries

Middle Back Strains

If you look at the back of most slim folks, you'll notice a hollow space between the inner border of the scapula and the spine. That's not supposed to be hollow! There are some very important muscles there that are responsible for moving the shoulder out, as in a tennis backstroke, and also holding our shoulders up to keep us from being round-shouldered (kyphosis or Dowager's Hump). Most people, not just skinny folks, have paper-thin muscles instead of the thick bands that allow us to move and stand correctly.

The three groups of muscles involved here are the middle fibers of the Trapezius, and two Rhomboids, the Major and Minor above it. In all of training, these are likely, the most neglected muscles of the upper body. Why? Because you can't see them. Most folks don't even know anything is there until they tear them. These muscles are the bane of racquet sportsmen.

Wielding a heavy racquet which must absorb the shock of an object striking it hard enough to change direction causes a lot of pressure on those weak little guys. When enough swings are executed and enough shock is absorbed, these muscles tear just like cloth. The initial tear is hard to make, but once it's started, it just keeps ripping easily. What's the trick to keep that from ever happening? Weights. Heavy weights and proper exercise.

What to do to recover:

- RICE
- Treatment for strain
- Restore range of motion through stretching
- Increase muscle mass and strength with weights

Levator Strains

There is one tiny overworked muscle between the top inner corner of the scapula and the back of your skull just behind the ears. This fellow is called the Levator Scapula. It is so prone to straining and spasm that many in physical medicine have nick named this guy "Darth Levator." Most of the time a pain in the back of your neck and upper back is caused by this guy. But it's not entirely his fault.

Since we were kids, we've been pitched forward looking at our meals in the high chair, working at desks in school or at the office, or sitting at shop tables or on assembly lines. Throughout all of this the poor Levator is on one hell of a stretch, yet we ask him to work holding our heads up! Then, when we get up from our stooped-over position, guess what – our heads and necks are still pitched forward and out of alignment with the spine, creating pressure on this small muscle. No wonder it goes on strike, tries to commit suicide, and tells us to fart off!

Look at the back of most people's necks. What do you see? Flab, string-like cords next to sunken hollows? Almost no one has a well-conditioned upper back and neck. This neglect coupled with over-work, leads to strains.

What to do to recover:

- RICE
- Treatment for strain
- Lift weights to increase muscle mass and strength
- Learn and practice proper posture when sitting, standing, and walking

The Shoulder Joint

The Shoulder Joint is entirely different from the AC or SC joints. Here, instead of a semi-movable joint, we have a fully movable ball and socket joint. In biomechanics the greater the range of motion, the shallower the joint. This leads to a propensity for dislocations and this joint can dislocate in 3 different directions! An external force is usually needed to force a shoulder out of its socket and stretch out the ligaments. Regardless of whether the ball (head) of the humerus goes down (inferior), pops out to the front (anterior), or gets shoved out behind (posterior), the result is the same: great pain, great spasm, immediate loss of function, and immediate onset of swelling which freezes the shoulder out of position. A shoulder joint dislocation mistreated or left out of position can severely injure the nerve bundle of the Brachial Plexus in the armpit. This can cause paralysis of the arm and shoulder. Don't monkey around with this one waiting for it to go away on it's own; it won't.

Unless you know how to relocate a dislocated shoulder joint, let a pro do it. Once the swelling sets in, it will take ice and about 50cc's of intravenous Valium to relax the muscles and knock the anxious patients out enough to pop the joint back in.

For many "Old Jocks," especially former gymnasts, constantly dislocating shoulders is a fact of life. The shoulders go out when pulling bags out of the trunk of a car, when reaching above the head with the palm face down, or when your loved one is hanging onto your arm walking. In these cases the ligaments are so stretched out that the ball of the humerus isn't even sitting right in the socket; it's hanging about half its way down and rotated to the front! With this type of dislocation, the patient learns how to easily relocate the joint, as there is little tension to hold it in any position.

Dislocations cause a buildup of scar tissue which in time, restricts range of motion. The adhesions must be overcome by a well-planned bout of stretching. The muscles will atrophy after injury and should be regenerated by weight training and strength building.

A word about exercise. Not all shoulder exercise is good. There are many common shoulder, chest, and upper back exercises that will do more harm than good and should not be performed by any lifter over the age of 27 (physiologically when old age begins)! The following exercises will destroy the rotator cuff muscles of the shoulder:

- Behind the neck Pulldown
- Behind the neck Shoulder Press
- Wide grip front Pulldown
- Full Range of Motion Bench Press.
- Machine Chest Fly's

Read the rehab section to learn the whys of the biomechanics involved and to discover exercises superior to those listed as taboo above.

What to do to recover:

- Get medical attention very, very pronto
- RICE
- Treatment for strain
- Treatment for sprain
- Rehab with weights and stretching

Surgical Neck Fractures

Thankfully, these are not a common occurrence in sports. When the upper arm bone does fracture, it does so most often through what is known as the surgical neck of the humerus. That slim neck just out from the ball is called by its name because it's the part of the bone that has to have surgery most often. Many of the shoulder muscles attach at this area, so shoulder dysfunction and muscular atrophy are quite common as a result of these breaks.

What to do to recover:

- Get medical attention
- RICE
- Treatment for fracture
- Treatment for strain
- Do not return to upper body training or play until cleared
- Restore ROM with stretching
- Restore muscle mass and strength with weights

Rotator Cuff Injuries

The rotator cuff is comprised of a series of muscles that surround the top of the humerus, front and back, and have the job of rotating the shoulder inward and outward. For example, outward rotation is like the movement when one cocks back to throw a spear. Inward rotation is the inward and downward movement as the spear is thrown. These muscles arise at the scapulae, as well as the front (anterior) and side (lateral) chest wall. There are more inward than outward rotators as it is more important to throw the spear strongly than to cock it back strongly. These small but very important muscles take an absolute beating during sports and training.

Pain reaching up, pain in pulling something back, pain and restriction in reaching up and back with the elbow bent, and pain and restriction in reaching up from behind your back are all signs of rotator cuff injury.

If the injury is serious enough, surgical repair may be needed. A word of warning here: most orthopedists are horrible at doing shoulder surgery. And to top things off, the more conservative orthoscopic surgery may not necessarily be better than open shoulder surgery. If a lot needs to be done, the closed orthoscope procedure may take too long, keeping the patient anesthetized sometimes up to 4 hours! Aside from that, there is only so much cleaning and fixing you can do through a little joint scope. The open surgeries take no longer than two hours, less usually, and the surgeon can not only see what is wrong faster, he can use a variety of things to repair, clean, and fix what may be wrong faster, better, and surer than the guy with the scope can. It is one of the only surgeries where the radical open is far better than the conservative closed procedure.

What to do to recover:

- Seek medical advice
- RICE
- Treatment for strain
- Rehab with stretching and weights

The Other Shoulder Muscles

Most everyone admires the guy or gal with well-developed, well-rounded shoulder muscles. The ones most often gawked at are the deltoid or 3-headed muscle that forms the cap of the shoulder. But under the delts are several important muscles that are unknown by most but important when dealing with injury. The most often injured of these unknown structures is the long head of the bicipital tendon. Biceps you say? Isn't that an arm muscle? Yes it is, but just where do you think it's attached? At the top of the shoulder just below the point of the AC joint.

Try this test. Hold your arm down at your side with your palm facing toward your front. Strum your thumb across the front (anterior) deltoid muscle at your opposite side. Push in deep. Feel a cord like tendon there? Dig in now! Hurts, doesn't it! Now follow that tendon up to where it attaches at the top lip of the Glenoid socket. That might hurt too.

If you do any or all the aforementioned forbidden exercises, especially after the age of 27 through 35, you're likely to have chronic pain there. If you swim, pitch, or garden, you will have pain there. To continue doing the things you love, you'll need to condition your muscles using non-injuring strength exercises, changing the mechanics of what you do to lessen the strain on the muscles. Remember, the degrees of injury we spoke about earlier in this book, if it hurts and has dysfunction for longer than a few minutes, it may be a second degree injury or greater. Get it evaluated; then get it rehabilitated.

What to do to recover:

- Evaluation by health professional to determine degree and extent of injury
- RICE
- Treatment for strain
- Rehabilitate and recondition with stretching and weights

Rehab for Shoulder Injuries

At the shoulder, little hurts feel like big hurts and big hurts are crippling. This area of the body is better fed with nerves than blood; therefore, injuries are felt more, atrophy faster, and heal slower than injuries elsewhere. Dislocations of the bones in the shoulder joint (upper arm and shoulder socket) and, the shoulder girdle (point of the shoulder just above the shoulder joint) are quite common, and once the dislocation has been resolved and rested, rehabilitative exercise needs to be done. The same is true for all strains of the musculature of the shoulder. Once rested they need to be made stronger than they were previously to better withstand the pressures of work and to overcome the weakness and loss of muscle mass that comes along with the injury!

Putting first things first, range of motion comes before strength, so for our at-home program, we'll stretch and then lift.

Supine Rotator Cuff Stretches

Lie face up on your bed. Have a 2 to 5 pound ankle weight secured around the wrist (or hold a weight in your hand). Use a lighter weight at first and as the range of motion increases and the pain of stretching lessons, make the weight slightly heavier as the weeks progress.

Hold your arm away from your body so that it is about 90 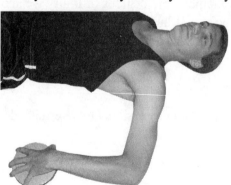 degrees from your side. Then bend the elbow to 90 degrees. Rotate the arm up toward your head and allow the arm to fall back of its own weight. Take it to the first point of pain and keep it there. This is external rotation. As you progress, the first point of pain will occur further and further into the stretch. Hold for 30 seconds.

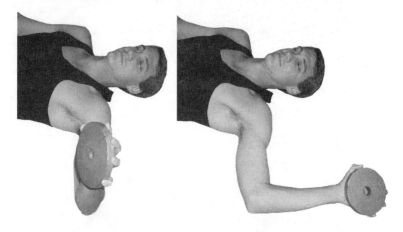

Then rotate your hand and arm toward your feet. Again, take it to the first point of pain and hold. This is internal rotation. Do each movement 4 times.

Standing Front Shoulder Stretch

Do essential stretch #4.

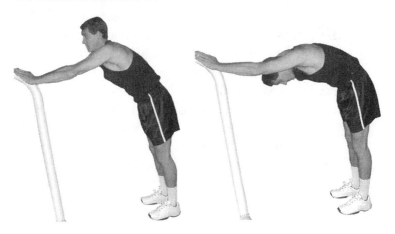

Now to getting the area stronger.

Single Dumbbell Upright Row

Stand with your feet slightly more than shoulder-width apart with knees slightly bent. From this stable position, have a

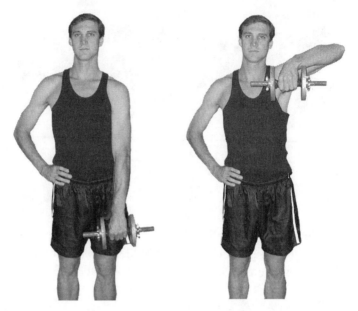

dumbbell in the hand on the affected side with as much weight as it will allow for some 7 repetitions. If you use a weight that is too light and add more repetitions, you will be gaining in endurance but not doing much to increase strength. Since most of our ADLs involve strength and not endurance, you won't be doing yourself any favors by babying yourself in rehab. Now draw the dumbbell up your side slowly, with your elbow out and away from you, until the bell is at mid-chest level. Do not hold but slowly allow the arm to return to its starting position. Take advantage of the resistance on the way down by moving slowly. This works the upper back, shoulder cap, and external rotator muscles. Do 3 sets of 5 to 7 repetitions.

External Rotation

Standing upright, hold your elbow. Rotate your arm using your elbow as a pivot so that your it moves from a 45 degree angle to

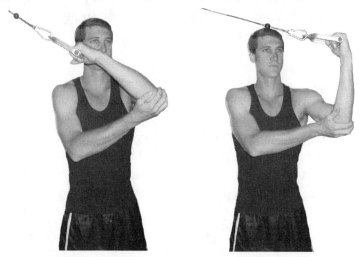

being up in line (90 degrees) with your ear. As you get stronger simply add more weight for resistance. Follow the guidelines stated earlier as to progression. Do 3 sets.

Internal Rotation

Using the same position as above only this time face away from the point of attachment. This time the hand begins by your ear at 90 degrees, then you will straighten the arm to 180 degrees. Three sets of 5 to 7 repetitions.

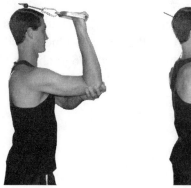
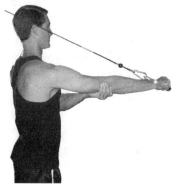

An often neglected area in the treatment of shoulder injuries are the muscles of the upper back. The superior fibers of the trapezius and the levator scapulae muscles are important as they elevate the shoulder in it's tasks and compensate for weaknesses and deficiencies in humeral abduction (bringing the arm out to the side away from the body).

Shoulder Shrugs

Stand as you did for the upright row. This stance balances you for work and stabilizes your lower back. Holding the dumbbell at arm's length, shrug the affected shoulder up toward your ear as if you were saying, "I don't know" but with only one side. 3 sets of 5 - 7 reps.

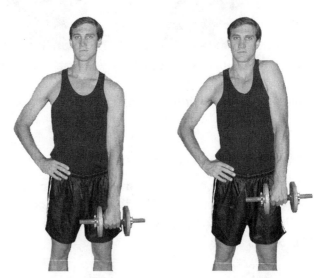

Shoulder exercise programs can get fancier, but this bare-bones basic one covers all of the bases. One baseball pitcher I rehabilitated went from not being able to abduct his arm much past 30 degrees to throwing a ball at 86 miles an hour in 3 months using this program.

Rehab for Mid Back Injuries

A chiropractor needs to be consulted to reduce the vertebral subluxations that will be present from a soft tissue injury to the mid back. The doctor can also put back any subluxed rib heads. The soft tissues need to be addressed next. As with the lumbars, the thoracic area needs to be strengthened and stretched. The muscles with the worst damage in this area always are the scapular stabilizers, i.e., the Rhomboids and the mid Trapezius. These structures draw our shoulder blades back toward each other. In most folks these muscles are nearly paper thin and very susceptible to injury. Ideally, the space between the shoulder blades should be filled with muscle; unfortunately, in most, the area is so underdeveloped and empty that you can place a hand in the hollow created by a lack of muscle. Muscle atrophy or underdevelopment there leads to rounded shoulders and overuse syndromes of the area such as frequent strains (muscle tears).

Just about any voluntary muscle reacts to injury by spasming. It's a muscle's way of freaking out. Spasm causes pain from the strength of the contraction and the lack of oxygenation that takes place during the spasm. Typically, during a muscular contraction, up to 80% of that muscle's blood supply is cut off. That's okay because most contractions are of short duration and the muscle works off of its own oxygen and sugar reserves. If the contraction continues after it's own O2 and glucose has been used up then a situation will happen that will be much like an experience we all had as kids.

Did you ever put rubber bands around your wrist to cut off the circulation to your hand? What happened? First, the hand turned an interesting shade of purple, then numb, and finally, the area began to throb and hurt. If you attempted to clench your fist at that time, you'll remember that it really hurt to do so. Well, in a spasm, after being contracted for so long with 80% of its oxygen cutoff and its metabolic wastes building up, you can understand why those hurt so much!

Stretching is the fastest self-help method to relieve a spasm. Stretching is literally forcing a muscle away from its shortening. It also has the added advantage of getting rid of adhesions. This is fibrotic scar tissue-like buildup that inhibits range of motion.

For those who can't touch their toes with the knees locked-adhesions cause a good bit of the burning pull you feel at the back of the thighs when you try to reach.

Essential Stretch #3 Beggars Stretch

Reach forward with one arm straight in front of you. Using the opposite hand, grasp the elbow on the extended side and draw that arm to the opposite shoulder. Keep the elbow straight and the palm face up. Have the stretched arm level or slightly above the opposite shoulder. Do not allow the shoulder on the side

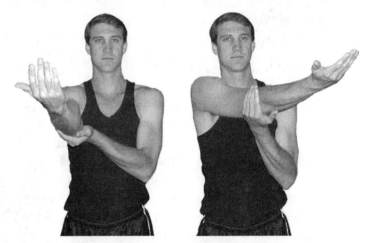

you're stretching to hike up. Press it down. Now drop your chin toward your chest to complete the stretch. Hurts so good doesn't it! Hold and count to 30. Bring the arm back, rest 10 seconds, and repeat. Do 4 stretches of 30 seconds duration per side.

Essential Stretch #4 Anterior Shoulder Stretch

The front of the shoulder is a chronically aching place for many folks. It is there that the overworked, overrotated, and under-stretched tendon called the Bicipital long-head lives. This longer tendon of the arm's bicep muscle helps to move the arm to the front and side and, with the help of the pectoral, moves the arm in toward the midline. Due to its placement in a shallow groove at the front of the arm bone, that it slips in and out of

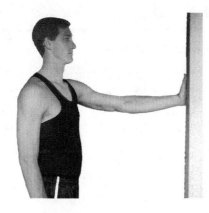

during shoulder movements, this tendon is one of the most painful in active folks over 35.

Place your hand on a wall at shoulder height with the fingertips pointed behind you. Leaving your hand fixed on the wall; turn toward the opposite arm. As with all stretches, take to the first point of mild pain and hold to a count of 30. Do each side 4 times for a 30-second count each.

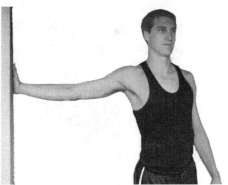

Mid and Upper Back Strengthening

Front Pulldown

Sit facing the machine and grasp the bar with your hands shoulder width apart and the palms facing you. This grip is the

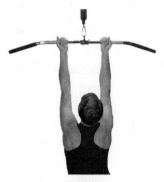

strongest position for movement in the torso. Pull the bar to just below your chin. Have a weight that initially won't allow you to do more than 7 repetitions. Breathe out when you pull and in when you return. Do 3 sets of 7 repetitions. Each week add one more repetition to each set until you hit 10 reps. That will take 4

weeks. Then, add 10 or 15 pounds to the stack and go back to doing 7 repetitions and work your way up the progression again.

Note: While this variation of the pulldown exercise is very sound and helpful, the palms away from you varieties are not! Those, especially the wide grip and behind the neck versions of the movement, do much damage to the front of the shoulder, aside from being inferior exercises due to lack of full ROM.

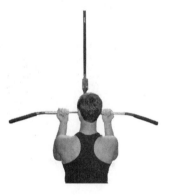

Seated Rowing

Sit upright with the knees slightly bent. Grasp a low pulley bar, palms down this time. From a straight arm position pull the bar to the bottom of your chest. As you pull, have your elbows out away from your body and think about bringing the shoulder blades together. Exhale as you pull. Set the weight using the recommendations described above and progress as described for 3 sets of 7 to 10 repetitions.

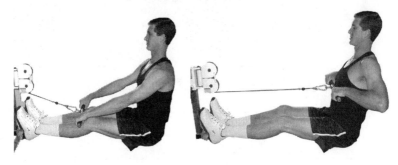

Bent Over Dumbbell Rows

Use a dumbbell that will allow for 7 repetitions. Kneel one knee on an exercise bench placing the same side hand on the bench as well. This will stabilize the back and reduce the stress on it.

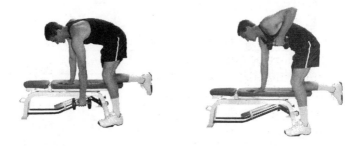

Grasping the dumbbell, bend at the waist with the weighted arm hanging down. Draw the dumbbell to the waist while breathing out. Do 3 sets of 7 to 10 repetitions. This exercise can be substituted for the seated rowing.

Resistance exercise should be done only 2 to 3 times a week.

NOTES

Chapter 12
Arm and Hand Injuries
● ● ● ● ● ●

Injuries to the upper extremities are usually straightforward because these structures are not weight-bearing, although there is some crossover since the tricep and bicep muscles connect at the shoulder joint. The lower extremity, the pelvis, and, the spine all bear with the weight and effort of the body. How they were hurt may not always be obvious but may need to be inferred from what the athlete was doing and how he was moving at the time. It is easier to determine how the arms sustained injury and, therefore it is easier to come to a correct diagnosis. An anatomical note is important here for a clearer understanding. In anatomy, the arm is not everything from the shoulder to the wrist; it is only that area from the shoulder to the elbow. The segment of the upper extremity below the elbow is called the forearm. Keep this distinction in mind as you read.

Most Common Injuries

Strains to the Bicep and Triceps Muscles

These two muscles are not the only ones in the arm, but they do comprise most of the muscular mass. While they can be strong, their weak points are their tendons. Remember, the tendons are the things that connect muscle to bone. They are cord-like structures that stretch somewhat but do not, themselves, contract. When faced with a load greater than they can handle, tears occur within the tendons themselves, or they are torn from the bone. A tear from the bone is an avulsion and may take a piece of bone with it when it happens.

As with all injuries the extent of the injury determines the corrective procedure. If the tear is light (1st degree), then RICE and nutrition will be enough to promote healing. Medium (2nd degree) strains will require care so that they do not fully tear. The resting time is longer, as is the healing, RICE, and nutrition period; some stretching and strengthening will need to be done. Full tears (3rd. Degree) need surgery to repair followed by an extensive period of restoring range of motion and strengthening. This must be coupled with proper nutritional treatment if the healing time is to be speeded up.

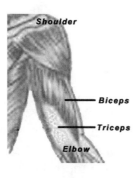

What to do to recover:

- RICE

- If there is longer than just momentary loss of function, strength and range of motion get the injury evaluated by an orthopedist or athletic trainer

- Treatment for strain

Bursitis of the Elbow

Injuries of the lower tricep tendon are oftentimes accompanied by an egg shaped swelling at the point of the elbow. This is known as Olecranon bursitis. This swollen bursa sack tends to be a persistent cuss and is difficult to get rig of even after the tendon is healed. Ice water baths where the elbow is immersed in a large salad bowl of ice water for 20 minutes are the preferred treatment. Compression bandages, elbow braces, and the like worn during the

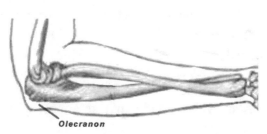

Olecranon

day, while at play or training, keep the area from further swelling and help to squeeze out effusion in the bursar sac.

What to do to recover:

- RICE
- Treatment for strain

Epichonditis (Tennis, Golf, and Pitcher's Elbows)

These are strains of the area directly above and to either side of the elbow where the muscles of the forearm attach to the lower end of the humerus. There is a ridge of coarse bone to the inside and outside of the lower humerus that acts as a perfect purchase for these tendons. When we move naturally, there is hardly any strain on these tendons but sports activities are contrived movement and not natural to the body. Let me explain.

When someone invents a sport or activity, they first conceive of its goal. For example: to hit a ball across a net so the other person can't hit it back or to kick a ball across a line passed those attempting to intercept the ball. You get the picture. The human body must conform to best achieve the goals of that game. No one in the western world has ever developed a movement form, from sport to dance, that ever first took into consideration the biomechanics of the human body. No, the body was made to conform to the sport instead of the sport conforming to the body. In the Far East the body was first made to move mimicing the motions of animals or the supposed actions of demigods. But, some two hundred years ago the monks at Shaolin figured out that making man move like man was the smartest and easiest way to move with great power, speed, and unbelievable steadiness. From that realization came Wing Chun, Pak Me, and Plum Blossom, the last martial artists to emerge from Shaolin.

Wrist Injuries

The wrist is a very mobile joint capable of flexion, extension, abduction, adduction, and circumduction. As such, it is a very

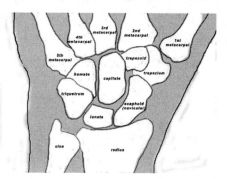

shallow joint comprised of the seven small cuneiform bones articulating with the ends of the forearm bones below and the carpal bones of the hand above.

Rehab for Upper Arm Injuries

Here we see the results mainly of strains, sprains and fractures. More serious injuries such as those caused by crushing or that result in amputation will not be dealt with here.

Range of motion in the upper arm is adversely affected by inactivity resulting from time spent in a splint or cast. The muscles that bend the elbow "set," becoming abnormally shortened (contractured). This need not be permanent, however. Passive stretching, assisted or unassisted, can restore full range of motion in just a few weeks. For those who must rehab themselves without much help from professionals, let me show you a simple way to stretch out a contractured elbow joint. If full range of motion is not achieved in a few months, then tissue will begin to build up on the joint, creating a restriction that only a surgeon will be able to reduce. You don't want that.

Passive Elbow Flexor Stretching

Sit and bend at the waist so that you can grasp a medium weight dumbbell with your affected side. Form a "v" between the knee on that side and the forearm of your opposite arm. Now tilt your body back and bring the elbow on the effected side up to the

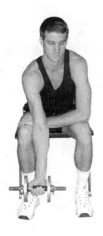 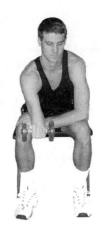

notch. Let the dumbbell hang and tug on the adhesions of the elbow. Hold this position for a full minute. If that is impossible, lighten the weight used so that a minute can be attained. Rest for a minute, then repeat the stretch another 3 times for a total of 4 reps. Do this daily.

Upper Arm Strengthening

Pick one curling exercise for the front of the arm and one extension exercise for the back.

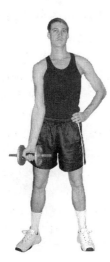

Dumbbell Curls

Using our shoulder width stance and slightly bent knees, hold a dumbbell on the affected side at arms length. With the palm facing up toward

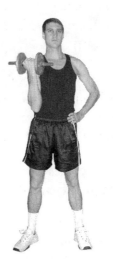

the ceiling, bend the elbow and arc the hand to the shoulder. Do 3 sets of 5 to 7 repetitions.

Concentration Curls

Using the same seated position as in the elbow stretch – keep the elbow nestled in the notch and bend it in order to bring the hand 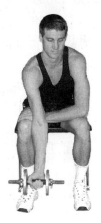 and the bell toward your face. Do 3 sets of 5 to 7 repetitions.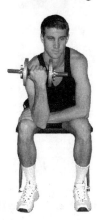

Rubber Band Tricep Extensions

With bungi cord firmly secured to a doorknob or other fixed object, lean forward bracing the hand of the non – affected side on the knee. Hold the elbow on the affected side by the ribs and have the arm bent to 90 degrees. Pull back against the cord to straighten out the elbow for 3 sets of 5 to 7 repetitions. As the

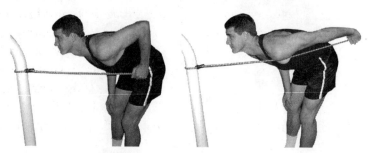

resistance becomes easier, move back further from the point of attachment to increase the tension of the cord.

Standing Dumbbell Tricep Extension

Stand with feet slightly more than shoulder width apart, knees slightly bent. Grasp the dumbbell with the affected side and

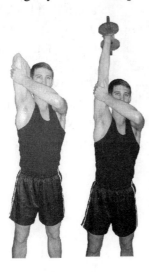

raise the weight over your head. Holding the elbow at ear level, have the elbow bent and the dumbbell behind your head. Begin the movement by straightening the arm so that the weight moves overhead. Do 3 sets of 5 to 7 repetitions. If you are using an adjustable dumbbell, be sure that the collars are on tightly as you don't want the weights to come loose while you're working with them above your head.

Rehab for Forearm and Wrist Injuries

Here we have an area capable of several different motions most of which need to be addressed in our stretching and strengthening program. First of all, let me say that as a society of power steering button pushers we have nowhere near the forearm and wrist strength our agricultural and early industrial age ancestors had. It has definitely been a case of didn't use it – lost it. Anatomists have discovered that most of western man has lost a muscle in the forearm and one at the back of the upper arm – all from non-use. The goal for folks whose work concentrates effort at the hand, wrist, and forearm is to build strong sinewy flexible muscles here.

Wrist Extension Stretch

Hold your arm ahead of you, with the hand and wrist held as if you were pushing something away. Grasp the hand on that side

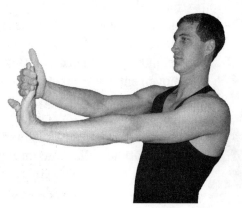

and pull it back toward you. As always, take the stretch to the first point of pain and hold it for 30 seconds; then rest. Do a total of 4 stretches in this direction.

Wrist Flexion Stretch

Hold your arm as above, but this time bend the wrist so the hand is pointing down. Holding by the knuckles, press the hand gently in toward you and stretch. Do 4 times for 30 second each.

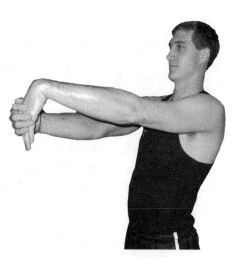

Wrist Adduction Stretch

With the arm ahead of you again, have your palm face into your midline as shown. Grasp the hand and gently pull the fingers toward the floor. Hold at the first point of pain. Repeat for a total of 4 repetitions.

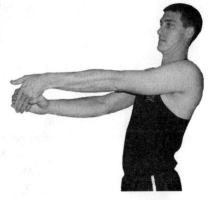

Lower Arm Strengthening

School Bell Ringing Exercise (Lateral flexion of the wrist)

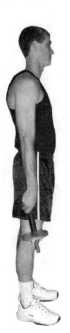

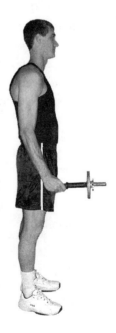

This excellent exercise for outside tennis elbow (lateral epicondylitis) and hand and wrist weakness can be performed with a small sledge hammer (3 lbs.) or a dumbbell bar with the weight only on one side. Hold the hammer or dumbbell by the unweighted end. Have your arm at your side with your elbow locked. Starting with the hammer pointing toward the ground, tip the head up toward the ceiling using only your wrist. Do not bend the elbow or turn the wrist to help. Do 3 sets of 5 to 7 reps.

Reverse School Bell Ringing (Medial Flexion of the Wrist)

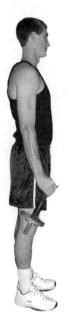

This time we hold the weighted end behind us with the arm in the same position. With the weight pointed toward the floor, tip the head up toward the ceiling by moving the wrist. You will find that you are stronger in this movement than in the one before. This is because you've got more muscles working in this direction than in the other. Complete 3 sets of 5 to 7 repetitions.

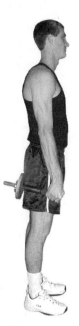

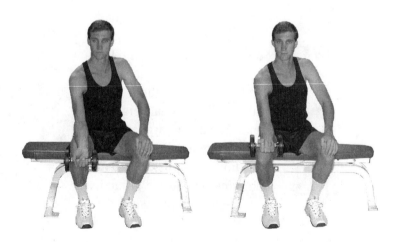

Wrist curls (Anterior Flexion)

Sit and have your forearm draped, palm up, on your lap. Hang your hand over the knee and grasping the dumbbell, curl the hand up toward the ceiling against the weight for 3 sets of 5 to 7 repetitions.

Reverse Wrist Curls (Posterior Flexion)

Same starting position as above only this time your palm is facing the floor. Curl the weight up and bring the knuckles back toward you. Do 3 sets of 5 to 7 repetitions. Avoid the urge to

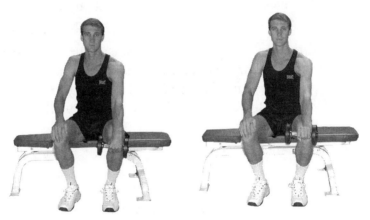

straighten the elbow by keeping the forearm flat against the thigh.

Hammer Curls

Stand with feet shoulder-width apart and knees slightly bent. Hold a dumbbell down at arms length on the affected side with the palm side of the hand turned in toward

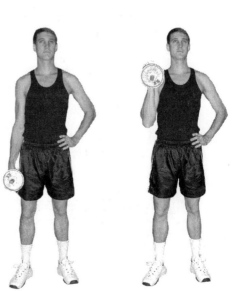

the side of the thigh. Bend the elbow and curl the weight to the shoulder while maintaining the hand position. Do 3 sets of 5 to 7 repetitions.

This series of exercises for the forearm and wrist are extensive but, again, given the different structures, motions, and uses of the forearm and wrist, all this work is needed.

The question often arises, "Do I work out both limbs or only the injured one?" After an injury, we tend to have residual weakness and atrophy on the affected side. This puts that side out of balance with the extremity that is not injured. It's important that the injured limb first re-acquire the strength of the non-injured side; then both sides can be exercised together.

After you've recovered from your injury, it is important to continue with your stretching and strengthening work. Most important to the maintenance of flexibility in the frame are the stretches titled "essential": and these should be done daily for life.

NOTES

NOTES

Chapter 13
Head, Face, and Neck Injuries
• • • • • •

I've purposely left this chapter out. There are no injuries to these sensitive areas that I would call self-help injuries. Whenever these areas are hurt, get medical attention fast – remember any degree of concussion can kill. 'Nuff said

• • • • • •

Chapter 14
Treatments and Nutritional Maintenance
••••••

This chapter provides the treatments referenced in Chapters 7 through 12 under the heading "What to do to recover" for each of the common injuries. General nutritional maintenance guidelines are also discussed.

The treatments included are:

- Treatment for Sprains
- Treatment for Strains
- Treatment for Fractures
- Treatment for Contusion or Hemorrhage
- Treatment for Bone Spurs and Arthritis
- Treatment for Inflammation
- Treatment for Post-operative Recovery

Dr. William Wong, N.D.,PhD

Treatment for Sprains

Systemic Enzymes:
  5 to 10 tablets or capsules 3 times daily
Glucosamine / MSM supplement:
  4 tablets daily
Ice application:
  20 minutes - 1 to 2 times daily
Drawing Ointment:
  Apply lightly over contusion site 2 to 3
  times daily
Compression Braces with Support:
  Do not use elastic bandages

Dr. William Wong, N.D.,PhD

Treatment for Strains

Systemic Enzymes:
  5 to 10 tablets or capsules 3 times daily
Protein:
  1 gm per kilo of bodyweight daily
Zinc:
  50 to 100 mg daily
Vitamin E:
  800 IU daily
Vitamin A:
  10.000 IU daily
Androstene Cream:
  Men - 2 to 3 applications daily
  Women - 1 application daily

Dr. William Wong, N.D.,PhD

Treatment for Fractures

Systemic Enzymes:
  5 to 10 tablets or capsules 3 times daily
Calcium / Magnesium, Vitamin D supplement:
  2 tablets daily
Magnesium:
  Extra 1000 mg daily
Glucosamine / MSM supplement:
  2 tablets daily
Zinc:
  50 to 100 mg daily
Vitamin D:
  400 IU daily
Androstene Cream:
  Men - 2 applications daily
  Women - 1 application daily

Dr. William Wong, N.D.,PhD

Treatment for Contusion or Hemorrahage

Systemic Enzymes:
  5 to 10 tablets or capsules 3 times daily
Sublingual B 12 supplement:
  One eyedropper full daily
Iron Tonic:
  One tablespoon daily
Zinc:
  50 to 100 mg daily
Vitamin E:
  800 IU daily
Protein:
  1 gram per kilo of bodyweight daily
Vitamin C:
  1000 to 2000 mg daily
Rutin:
  1000 mg daily
Drawing Ointment:
  Apply lightly over contusion site 2 to 3
  times daily

Dr. William Wong, N.D.,PhD

Treatment for Bone Spurs and Arthritis

Systemic Enzymes:
  5 to 10 tablets or capsules 3 times daily
Glucosamine / MSM supplement:
  4 tablets daily
Magnesium:
  2000 mg daily
Vitamin B 6:
  100 mg daily
Vitamin E:
  800 mg daily

Dr. William Wong, N.D.,PhD

Treatment for Inflammation

Systemic Enzymes:
   10 tablets or capsules 2 to 3 times daily
Glucosamine / MSM supplement:
   4 tablets daily
Magnesium:
   2000 mg daily
Potassium:
   1000 mg daily

   (If measured as elemental potassium, take 198 mg daily.
   Each 99 mg of elemental potassium equals 500 mg of
   potassium.)

Drawing Ointment:
   Apply 2 to 3 times daily to inflammation

Dr. William Wong, N.D.,PhD

Treatment for Post-operative Recovery

Systemic Enzymes:
  5 tablets or capsules 3 times daily. Do what the European surgeons recommend: begin taking the enzymes 2 days postop if there are no excessive bleeding problems. These will prevent the build-up of post surgical scar tissue, speed healing, and reduce inflammation. Maintain this intake for at least 6 months.

Zinc:
  50 to 100 mg daily

Vitamin E:
  800 IU daily

Vitamin A:
  10.000 IU daily

Arthitol ES:
  4 tablets daily

Cal Guard:
  2 tablets daily

General Nutritional Maintenance

Remember general nutritional maintenance during recovery and rehabilitation. This includes the use of a complete vitamin mineral supplement; use a vitamin / mineral / essential nutrient powder. Plus, make sure you eat one gram of high grade protein per every 2.2 pounds of bodyweight. More than that can cause kidney stones and damage by greatly increasing the ammonia load the kidneys have to deal with as the unused protein does not go into building tissue but goes out in the urine.

Note: When combining two or more of the recommended treatments and the same supplement is recommended for both, do not take a double dose. Use the recommended dose for one. In other words, if combining the treatment plans for strains and fractures and both recommend systemic enzymes, take only 5 to 10 tablets 3 times a day total, <u>NOT</u> 5 to 10 for the strain and then 5 to 10 again for the fracture.